FAITH CURES, AND ANSWERS TO PRAYER

Women and Gender in North American Religions

Amanda Porterfield *and* Mary Farrell Bednarowski, *Series Editors*

FAITH CURES,

AND

ANSWERS TO PRAYER

Mrs. EDWARD MIX

WITH A CRITICAL INTRODUCTION BY
ROSEMARY D. GOODEN

SYRACUSE UNIVERSITY PRESS

The paper used in this publication meets the minimum requirements of American National Standard for Information Sciences—Permanence of Paper for Printed Library Materials, ANSI Z39.48–1984∞™

Library of Congress Cataloging-in-Publication Data

Mix, Edward, Mrs., 1832–1884.
Faith cures and answers to prayer / Mrs. Edward Mix ; with a critical introduction by Rosemary D. Gooden.— 1st ed.
p. cm. — (Women and gender in North American religions)
Originally published: Springfield, Mass. : Press of Springfield Printing Co., 1882. With new introd.
Includes bibliographical references.
ISBN 0-8156-2932-X (alk. paper)
1. Spiritual healing. I. Title. II. Series.
BR115.H4 M58 2002
234'.131—dc21
2002002050

Manufactured in the United States of America

For Jerry

Rosemary D. Gooden received her Ph.D. in American Studies from the University of Michigan. She lives in Chicago, Illinois.

CONTENTS

ACKNOWLEDGMENTS

MANY people have helped me in completing this project, and I am happy to acknowledge their contributions.

I would like to thank Amanda Porterfield for her enthusiastic support of this reprint. I also wish to thank her and Mary Farrell Bednarowski for reading my introductory essay and offering useful critical feedback. Words of thanks are inadequate to express my appreciation to Nancy Hardesty. She read my introduction and offered helpful criticism and insights, willingly shared her unpublished essays and valuable information from her research, and was a source of unwavering enthusiasm and support. My very sincere appreciation, too, to David Daniels, who read a portion of my essay, for his helpful suggestions and encouragement. Most of all, I thank him for introducing me to Sarah Mix.

I owe a special debt of gratitude to Meredith Kline and Freeman Barton of the Goddard Library of Gordon-Conwell Theological Seminary for their assistance and for granting permission for the use of the library's copy of *Faith Cures, and Answers to Prayer* for this reprint edition. I also thank Lynn Anderson of the Assemblies of God Archives for assistance. I am grateful to Jen Stegen and Ursula Scholz of the interlibrary loan department of Loyola University in Chicago for responding graciously and efficiently to my numerous requests. Gail Kruppa, archivist at the Torrington Historical Society, deserves special thanks for her responses to my inquiries and for sending me material on Sarah Mix.

I am grateful to the editors and other staff members at Syracuse University Press. It has been a pleasure to work with them. Special thanks are due Mary Selden Evans, executive editor, for her enthusiasm and support of this project. I want to thank Robert Mandel for his interest in and support of this reprint of *Faith Cures, and Answers to Prayer;* I also thank Jill Root, copy editor, and Lynn Hoppel of the marketing department for their excellent work.

I thank my family and friends for their interest in Sarah Mix and for their encouragement and support. My parents, Isaac and Mary Alice Gooden, were my staunchest supporters and always demonstrated confidence in me. My father died at the beginning of this project, and my mother toward the end of it, in the summer of 2001. I am saddened that they did not live to see its completion. I hope that I have honored them through my work on Sarah Mix.

It is difficult to find words to express my appreciation to my husband, Jerry DeMuth. He has lovingly supported me from the proposal stage to the final proofing. I thank him for his questions and comments on my drafts, for photocopying part of Mix's book while on a business trip in New York, and for keeping me sane and in good health with delicious gourmet meals during the completion of this project. This book is dedicated to him with my deepest love and gratitude.

PREFACE

SARAH Ann Freeman Mix (1832–1884), a free black woman who lived in Torrington, Connecticut, is a fascinating and important historical figure, a pioneer in the late-nineteenth-century divine healing, or faith healing, movement in America. A significant phenomenon in American religious history, faith healing involved praying for the miraculous cure of the sick. Sarah Mix was the first known African American healing evangelist and the first woman known to have made faith healing a full-time ministry. Countless sick women and men, and a few children, found healing through her prayer of faith and the laying on of hands. She was also a highly respected teacher, preacher, and writer. Carrie Judd Montgomery, who also became a prominent healing evangelist, writer, and teacher, found healing from a debilitating illness through Sarah Mix, whose healing ministry had been reported in a local newspaper. Mix's pioneering role in the divine healing movement, moreover, paved the way not only for Carrie Judd Montgomery, but also for Maria B. Woodworth-Etter and Aimee Semple McPherson, well-known twentieth-century evangelists whose ministries included healing. Even James Buckley, a prolific religious editor and formidable critic of the divine healing movement, noted Mix's prominence and respect as a faith healing practitioner.

Sarah Mix published and edited a journal on faith healing and wrote her spiritual autobiography. In 1882 she published *Faith Cures, And Answers to Prayer*, which includes an account of her healing, healing testimonials, and newspaper accounts of her ministry as a healing evangelist. This is the first reprint since its publication in 1882.

After nearly three decades of research and scholarship

devoted to the recovery of the religious history of American women, Sarah Mix is almost invisible in the historical record, her life and ministry unrecognized and nearly lost. Only recently has she been introduced to a wide audience and in a broader context. Nancy Hardesty included letters exchanged between Mix and Carrie Judd Montgomery in her chapter on evangelical women in *In Our Own Voices: Four Centuries of American Women's Religious Writing.*[1] Even more unknown are Mix's writings, which have been buried and unavailable. In fact, I did not learn of Mix's autobiography, *The Life of Mrs. Edward Mix, Written By Herself,* and the journal she founded and published, until I neared the end of my research for this introduction. Like works by other African American women, *Faith Cures, and Answers to Prayer* is available in only a handful of libraries. And there is only one known extant original copy of her autobiography. Because of the important information it provides about her life, *The Life of Mrs. Edward Mix, Written By Herself* is included as an appendix. This text is from a photocopy and, unfortunately, does not include Mix's photograph, which could not be reproduced for this publication.

In recent works on American religion, African American religion, and women's history, Sarah Mix's voice is silent. When Mix is mentioned in studies of faith healing, it is solely in relationship to her healing prayer for Carrie Judd Montgomery. While it is important to affirm the ministry of such an important figure in the divine healing movement as Carrie Judd Montgomery, it is equally important to acknowledge the central role of Sarah Mix, which deserves more recognition and study.

I believe that an important reason for Mix's absence from the historical record is that her ministry and life have been overshadowed by more well-known nineteenth-century female preachers and evangelists, black and white, including Amanda Berry Smith, Jarena Lee, Zilpha Elaw, Julia A. J. Foote and, most importantly,

Carrie Judd Montgomery. Another reason Sarah Mix's voice has been silent is that there simply is not a lot of information available on her. Short of a miraculous appearance of copies of her journal and other sources an historian would need, one can only dream about a sustained, critical examination of Mix's life and ministry. Additionally, most studies of African American women's religious experience have examined their experience within the context of the independent black denominations.[2] The historical record is fragmentary regarding black women's participation in the Holiness movement, Methodism, and the divine healing movement. I also believe there may exist an attitude and approach to black women's religious history that is similar to those demonstrated toward African American women writers, specifically, reading about black women's lives and varied experiences solely from the perspectives of the most popular writers. In the case of black women's religious history, Amanda Berry Smith, Jarena Lee, and others have become well-known. And it is important to know about them. But, as literary historian Nellie Mckay has stated, readers must "be aware of and interrogate the politics of silencing, erasure, and voice."[3] The same can be said for black women's religious experience. This reprint edition of *Faith Cures, and Answers to Prayer* is an attempt to fill important lacunae in black women's religious history and, more broadly, in the history of women and American religion.

The careers of nineteenth-century black women preachers and their varied texts have received scholarly attention by historians of women and religion, feminist critics, womanist theologians, and literary historians. Historians of religion and women's experience have benefited especially from the prodigious scholarship of literary historians, who have unearthed numerous texts written by nineteenth-century African American women that illuminate their religious experience. William Andrews' *Sisters of the Spirit: Three Black Women's Autobiographies of the*

Nineteenth Century was the first such anthology to emphasize
the religious experience of black women, namely Jarena Lee,
Zilpha Elaw, and Julia A. J. Foote.[4] And because of Henry Louis
Gates, Jr., general editor of the Schomburg Library of Nineteenth-Century Black Women Writers, the religious lives and
writings of Amanda Berry Smith, Katherine Davis Chapman Till-
man, Virginia Broughton, and Maria W. Stewart, to name a few,
have been brought to light.[5] In my search to find Mix in recent literary reference works and anthologies, I found Mrs. Edward
Mix listed in only one work: *Women Writers in the United
States: A Timeline of Literary, Cultural, and Social History* by
Cynthia J. Davis and Kathryn West.[6] The religious experiences
of countless other black women and their writings about those
experiences, needless to say, await excavation. This reprint edition of *Faith Cures, and Answers to Prayer* is a contribution to
the ongoing excavation of texts written by black women in the
nineteenth century. It introduces Mrs. Edward Mix to a wider
audience while, at the same time, highlighting her ministry in
the divine healing movement.

Finally, and most importantly, *Faith Cures, and Answers to
Prayer* is an effort to highlight the pioneering role of Sarah Mix
in the nineteenth-century divine healing movement and recast
the discussion of this critical period in American religious history through a closer look at her life and ministry. I hope that
readers will be as excited as I was to discover Sarah Mix, and
that making Mix and her ministry known will not only illuminate
the divine healing movement but also contribute to a deeper historical understanding of American religion, African American
religion, and, most importantly, African American women and
religion. Additionally, I hope this book will help to provide an
historical context in which to understand the current interest in
spirituality and health and the role of prayer and religious faith
in the healing of the body.

My introduction is divided into five sections. After briefly introducing her, the first section contextualizes the life and ministry of Sarah Mix through an historical overview of the Holiness and divine healing movements. The second section examines Sarah Mix's healing ministry within the broader historical continuum of African American healing traditions and the healing work of African American women. The third section provides a biographical sketch of Mrs. Edward Mix. The fourth section highlights *Faith Cures, and Answers to Prayer* and assesses the impact of Sarah Mix on the divine healing movement in America; an epilogue briefly notes the laying on of hands today.

My essay does not set out to provide a critique of the literary merits of *Faith Cures, and Answers to Prayer.* Nor does it evaluate the belief in miraculous cures. Rather, this essay places Sarah Mix in historical perspective. Her extraordinary life and ministry are central to the story of the divine healing movement in nineteenth-century America.

Notes

1. Nancy A. Hardesty, "Evangelical Women," in *In Our Own Voices: Four Centuries of American Women's Religious Writing*, ed. Rosemary Skinner Keller and Rosemary Radford Ruether (New York: HarperSanFrancisco, 1995), 232–33.

2. Presently, the best monograph on African American women's religious experience is Evelyn Brooks Higginbotham, *Righteous Discontent: The Women's Movement in the Black Baptist Church, 1880–1920* (Cambridge, Mass.: Harvard Univ. Press, 1993). An excellent historiographical overview of African American religion that includes African American women's religious experience is Judith Weisenfeld, "On Jordan's Stormy Banks: Margins, Center, and Bridges in African American Religious History," in *New Directions in American Religious History*, ed. Harry S. Stout and D. G. Hart (New York: Oxford Univ. Press, 1997), 414–44.

3. Nellie Y. McKay, "Beyond the Story: Reading Black Women's Lives in Madison, Wisconsin," *Women's Studies Quarterly* (1993): 164–71.

4. William L. Andrews, ed., *Sisters of the Spirit: Three Black Women's Autobiographies of the Nineteenth Century* (Bloomington: Indiana Univ. Press, 1986).

5. See, for example, Henry Louis Gates, Jr., ed., *Spiritual Narratives* (New York: Oxford Univ. Press, 1988).

6. Cynthia J. Davis and Kathryn West, *Women Writers in the United States: A Timeline of Literary, Cultural, and Social History* (New York: Oxford Univ. Press, 1996).

INTRODUCTION

SARAH MIX, Healing Evangelist

I was about to give up in despair, when I heard of the wonderful cures performed through Mrs. Mix. I sent for her to come and see me; when she came into the room she asked if I had faith to be healed. I told her I had perfect faith; she then anointed me and laid hands on me, all the while praying to God to heal me. I prayed with her, and our prayers were answered, for in less than an hour after she began to labor with me I got up, dressed, and walked out into the other room as well as anybody, perfectly free from pain and all my lameness gone . . . I am still gaining strength fast and feel well. I would add that all sufferers who may see this *may* have faith in God. Send for Mrs. Mix and be cured.

—MRS. G. A. WILTON[1]

SARAH Ann Freeman Mix (1832–1884), known in her ministry as Mrs. Edward Mix, was the first known African American healing evangelist in the United States and the first known female to have a full-time healing ministry.[2] One of the pioneers of the divine healing movement, Mix was a well-known advocate and practitioner of faith healing.[3] Both the religious and secular press reported Mix's ministry, which was so successful that physicians referred patients to her. An itinerant evangelist, she traveled primarily throughout New England and, at the same time, extended her healing ministry through correspondence by writing letters of support and encouragement to individuals who were healed through her ministry. With her husband,

Edward, a "religious worker" and frequent traveling companion, Sarah Mix also maintained a "faith home" in their Torrington, Connecticut, residence.[4] In addition, she conducted a weekly Wednesday prayer meeting there for women.

A prolific religious writer, Sarah Mix was editor and publisher of *Victory Through Faith*, a monthly journal on faith healing. Additionally she wrote an eight-page leaflet, *In God We Trust*, and contributed articles on faith healing to *Triumphs of Faith*, the journal founded by Carrie Judd (later known as Carrie Judd Montgomery).[5] In 1882 Sarah Mix published *Faith Cures, and Answers to Prayer*, one of two books she wrote. It includes an account of her healing from consumption through the ministry of Ethan Otis Allen, who was regarded as the "father of divine healing"; a compilation of testimonies from people healed through Mix's prayers; newspaper accounts of her healing ministry; and other testimonials and writings on faith healing.

Sarah Mix also wrote her autobiography, *The Life of Mrs. Edward Mix, Written By Herself*, in 1880. It was not published, however, until 1884, after her death that year.[6] Chronologically, Mix's spiritual autobiography begins with her birth and spans her early childhood through her ministry as a healing evangelist. Totaling only twenty-four pages, *The Life* includes a photograph of Mix as well as a six-page appendix written by her husband, Edward M. Mix. An invaluable source of information, Sarah Mix's personal narrative is the only known extant text that provides vital personal information about her life, including her childhood and young adulthood, her marriage, the loss of her children, and her healing. Most importantly, Mix's spiritual autobiography emphasizes the process of her religious conversion and her calling by God to "Go work in my vineyard," the impetus to her ministry as a healing evangelist.

The life and ministry of Sarah Mix can be more completely understood by examining the historical background of the divine healing movement, especially the Holiness movement, which played a critical role in the emergence of the divine healing movement in late-nineteenth-century America, its doctrine of Christian perfection providing a theological foundation for faith healing.

The Historical Context: From Christian Perfection to Faith Healing

Several events and individuals played a crucial role in the emergence of the divine healing movement in late-nineteenth-century America. Most notable among these was the emerging Holiness movement among evangelical Protestants that began in the 1830s as a revival in Methodism.[7] Although influenced by Methodists, the Holiness movement was interdenominational and included Baptists, Presbyterians, and Congregationalists among its earliest adherents. Returning to the views of John Wesley (1703–1791), the founder of Methodism, the early Holiness movement revived Wesley's teaching on and experience of "Christian Perfection." In his sermon "Christian Perfection" (1741) and *A Plain Account of Christian Perfection* (1766), Wesley taught that Christian perfection, synonymous with holiness, entire sanctification, and perfect love, was a second, instantaneous work of grace separate from conversion and received by faith. At the same time, Wesley believed that sanctification was a gradual process.[8]

Phoebe Palmer, Holiness Evangelist

Phoebe Worrall Palmer (1807–1874), a Methodist laywoman, was the best known and most influential leader of the Holiness movement and the most effective articulator of perfectionist doctrine.[9] Palmer reformulated Wesley's views with her concept

of a "shorter way," the belief that sanctification was an immediate experience, as opposed to a gradual process. Through her
"altar theology" Palmer taught that "laying all on the altar" was
the means to sanctification, or holiness. Christ was the altar that
sanctified the Christian's total dedication of self. Palmer, who
experienced entire sanctification in 1837, employed her "altar
theology" in her popular book, *The Way of Holiness*, first published in 1843. From 1864 to 1874, the last decade of her life,
Palmer edited the journal *Guide to Holiness*, a leading Holiness
periodical.[10] Most important, from 1840 until her death thirty-
four years later, Palmer was the leader of the Tuesday Meeting
for the Promotion of Holiness.[11] The Tuesday Meeting, which
lasted more than sixty years, became the principal arena of the
Holiness movement in the Methodist Episcopal Church as well
as the center of Palmer's leadership in the Holiness movement.[12]
Although initially open only to women, men began attending in
1839, after Thomas C. Upham, a professor at Bowdoin College
whose wife, Phoebe, was a regular attender, asked if he could attend. Upham experienced entire sanctification, and soon prominent Methodist bishops, ministers, theologians, and educators
began attending. By the 1850s the Tuesday Meeting included
laity and clergy from most Protestant denominations.[13] The
well-known African American Holiness evangelist Amanda
Berry Smith (1837–1915) occasionally attended the Tuesday
Meeting.[14]

The preeminent religious leadership of Phoebe Palmer was
crucial to the growth of the Holiness movement. She helped
shape Holiness theology through her "altar theology" and taught
that publicly testifying to one's experience of holiness was necessary for retaining that experience. Palmer, moreover, built
upon one of Charles Finney's "new measures" in affirmning
women's public testimony.[15] Over time, according to Jean Miller
Schmidt, these two contributions by Palmer distinguished the

Holiness movement. Along with the theological system Palmer developed, her emphasis on public testimony provided women with a pronounced leadership role and with the opportunity for public ministry in the Holiness movement.[16] Women were also able to have major roles in the development of Holiness denominations. Most importantly, Phoebe Palmer, as a successful evangelist in the Holiness movement, influenced the lives of countless women, many of whom, like Sarah Mix, would also become evangelists.

The Holiness revival flourished in the camp meetings of the 1860s. These camp meetings were the primary means through which Holiness teaching was disseminated and, with the founding of the National Camp Meeting Association for the Promotion of Holiness in 1867, was further institutionalized. The movement's teaching was also disseminated through its publishing wing, the National Publishing Association for the Promotion of Holiness, which published numerous books and periodicals to promote holiness. Its main periodical, the *Christian Witness and Advocate of Bible Holiness*, which began publication in 1870, was published until 1959. In the 1870s and 1880s local, state, and regional organizations, along with several annual camp meetings in different locations, promoted Holiness teaching in the post-Civil War Holiness revival. By the end of the nineteenth century, the Holiness movement included numerous new publications on Holiness, various independent evangelistic and missionary movements, and new denominations, including the Christian and Missionary Alliance, the Church of God (Anderson, Indiana), and the Salvation Army.[17]

The Holiness movement provided a theological framework and methodology for the emergent divine healing movement. As Paul Chappell has pointed out, some of the distinctive features and practices of the Holiness movement were appropriated by the divine healing movement. These features and practices include interdenominationalism, special weekday services for healing similar to the Tuesday Meeting for the Promotion of Holiness, the use of the printed word to spread the doctrine of faith healing, and women's opportunity to have a public ministry. The divine healing and Holiness movements, moreover, shared basic beliefs, and healing evangelists' loyalties often lay with both movements.[18]

Ethan Otis Allen, Faith Healing Pioneer

Ethan O. Allen (1813–1902), a Methodist layman, was the first to formally link the Holiness doctrine of perfection to faith healing. In 1846 he experienced both sanctification and healing from consumption through prayer and the laying on of hands by Methodist class leaders. Divine healing was not a standard practice among American Methodists. John Wesley had practiced healing through prayer, although this was not the focus of his ministry.[19] Believing that purification from sin through sanctification would eradicate sickness, Allen went on to become the first itinerant evangelist to make faith healing a full-time ministry. Although divine healing was central to his ministry, Allen generated a fourfold doctrinal statement that, in addition to divine healing, included salvation, sanctification, and premillennialism. In his fifty-year ministry, primarily to the "disinherited of society," Allen traveled throughout the Northeast and New England to pray, usually one-on-one, with the sick in their homes, at camp meetings, and, as they were established, in faith cure homes. Allen prayed for poor sick people who had a variety of complaints as well as epileptics, the insane, and the incurable.[20]

Allen based his practice on Mark 16:17–18: "And these signs will accompany those who believe: by my name they will . . . lay their hands on the sick, and they will recover" (New Revised

Standard Version [NRSV]). His method was simple. Emphasizing the importance of believing with a sense of expectation, Allen prayed for the sick, whom he expected to be healed instantaneously. This expectation corresponded to the Holiness belief that perfection occurred instantaneously. Because he believed that the use of medicine as well as medical care by a physician indicated a lack of faith and trust in God, Allen did not commend either to those seeking bodily healing through prayer. Traveling companions, or "assistants," often accompanied Allen on his visits to the sick. Although Allen had at least two male traveling companions, it appears that more women than men aided Allen in his ministry.[21] Allen helped Sarah Mix find healing from consumption and, after helping her discern her vocation as a healing evangelist, she became one of Allen's earliest assistants. Mix and her husband, Edward, traveled with Allen before beginning their own faith healing ministry.[22]

Charles Cullis, W. E. Boardman,
A. B. Simpson, and A. J. Gordon

The divine healing movement in America, also referred to as "faith healing," "faith cure," or simply "healing movement," like the Holiness movement, became a significant phenomenon in American religion and culture beginning in the 1870s. Its proponents and practitioners believed that scriptural passages that promised healing, especially the promise of Jesus in Mark 16:18 and the promise of healing through "the prayer of faith" in James 5:14–15, were available to every generation of believers. In the 1870s Charles Cullis, W. E. Boardman, A. B. Simpson, and A. J. Gordon, proponents of Christian perfection who were actively involved in the Holiness movement, began systematically teaching and practicing faith healing and, by the 1880s, were among its most prominent practitioners and apologists.[23]

Charles Cullis (1833–1892), an Episcopal layman and homeopathic physician in Boston, like Ethan O. Allen was an important bridge between the Holiness and faith healing movements. Cullis persuaded prominent Holiness leaders that complete salvation included both spiritual and physical healing. He also adapted methods of the Holiness movement, such as the camp meeting, to promote faith healing and at the same time developed new ones such as the faith convention, an institution that would become integral to the late-nineteenth-century divine healing movement. Cullis was unique among the movement's leaders in America: As a layman he was influential and successful in the growth of the divine healing movement; as a physician, he maintained his medical practice while advocating faith healing.

In 1862 Cullis, who had attended Phoebe Palmer's Tuesday Meeting, claimed the experience of sanctification and believed that God was calling him to a "special work." In Boston in 1864 he commenced his "Faith Work," the name he gave his newfound ministry, by opening a home for consumptives. The ministry expanded to include additional homes for consumptives, an orphanage, a deaconess school, a faith training college, a chapel, and a publishing house, the Willard Tract Repository, founded in 1868. Additionally, Cullis's Faith Work included the Boydton Institute, a college and orphanage for blacks in the South; an evangelistic outreach to both blacks and Chinese immigrants; and missionary work in India and South Africa. Cullis also held Tuesday consecration, or holiness, meetings.[24]

Faith healing became a central focus of Cullis's Faith Work in the early 1870s, a result of his conviction that James 5:14–15 was true and applicable for his time. Cullis was also influenced by the work of European faith healers, especially the faith work of Dorothea Trudel in Mannedorf, Switzerland. Cullis had read her autobiography and was convinced that God could perform physical healings in Boston just as he was doing in Switzerland. Cullis became even more convinced of the efficacy of "the prayer of faith" when his patient Lucy Drake was healed of a brain tumor three months after he anointed her with oil and prayed for her.[25] After visiting Dorothea Trudel's faith work in Mannedorf in the summer of 1873, Cullis returned to Boston with a renewed zeal for faith healing and publicly acknowledged, for the first time, his call by God to a faith healing ministry.

In 1874 Cullis convened his first annual "Faith Convention," or camp meeting, in Framingham, Massachusetts. Beginning in 1876, conventions were held at Old Orchard Beach, Maine, where they continued until 1884, when Cullis purchased his own site at Intervale, New Hampshire.[26] Daily preaching services emphasized salvation and holiness and only one faith healing service was held, usually at the end of the convention. During this service several hundred individuals approached the altar for prayer and anointing with oil by Cullis. Many claimed instantaneous healing, whereas others believed their health would be restored gradually by faith. Those who sought the healing prayers of Cullis, either at his faith home or at faith conventions, reported having been sick for a long time and that medicine and care by a physician had been ineffective in producing a cure or restoration of health. As Cullis noted in his annual reports, common illnesses for which healing prayer was sought included cancer, chronic rheumatism, consumption, and paralysis.

The faith conventions were important to promoting the doctrine of faith healing and Cullis's healing ministry, as well as to the ministry of other healing practitioners. Cullis's faith conventions, especially the 1881 convention at Old Orchard Beach, generated enormous interest by the religious and secular presses. The number of extraordinary healings reported at the 1881 convention prompted increased attention by newspapers at the

1882 convention. As a result, faith healing received significant press coverage over the next few years.[27]

The printed word was as vital to spreading the doctrine of faith healing as it was to spreading the Holiness doctrine of Christian perfection. Testimonies, both oral and written, encouraged others to believe in God's promise regarding healing and to expect that they too would be healed. Because various branches and associations of the Holiness movement believed in the power of personal testimonies whereby one related one's experiences with God, compilations of healing testimonies were published in book form and as feature stories in faith healing periodicals.[28]

From 1872 to 1892 Cullis's Willard Tract Repository published nearly twenty major works and several tracts on faith healing, more than any other publisher in the United States. As a press, it inaugurated systematic publishing of works on divine healing, including three volumes by Cullis. These works were the first such testimonials of divine healing and the model for other books of healing testimonials. With the publication of Cullis's first book, *Faith Cures; or Answers to Prayer in the Healing of the Sick* (1879), both the doctrine of faith healing and Cullis's faith healing ministry gained widespread exposure.[29] In his study on the faith cure movement, Raymond Cunningham has argued: "Important as the annual Faith Conventions were, the Willard Tract Repository was perhaps even more so in making Cullis' Faith Work the focal point of faith cure interest in the United States." By the mid-1880s, the Repository had published seventeen titles on spiritual healing.[30]

Cullis's critical role in connecting Holiness and faith healing is also evident in his influence on such leading Holiness leaders as W. E. Boardman and A. B. Simpson. He convinced them of the scriptural basis of praying for the physical healing of the sick and of his belief that complete salvation included not just healing of the spirit but also healing of the body.[31] Both Boardman and Simpson went on to become influential leaders in the divine healing movement in the 1880s and, with A. J. Gordon, wrote important theological and doctrinal works defending faith healing.

W. E. Boardman (1810–1896), a Presbyterian minister and frequent attender of the Tuesday Meeting for the Promotion of Holiness, became a leader in the Holiness movement in 1859 when his book *The Higher Christian Life* was published. As an itinerant preacher, he conducted Holiness faith conventions for Charles Cullis. Boardman also wrote a series of articles on sanctification for Cullis's magazine, *Times of Refreshing*, beginning a literary partnership in which Cullis's Willard Tract Repository published several works by Boardman and Cullis's biography of Boardman. A close friend of Cullis, Boardman compiled Cullis's journals documenting the first eight years of his Faith Work, which were published as *Faith Work Under Dr. Cullis* in Boston in 1874 by the Repository.[32]

Boardman and Cullis together toured the faith homes of Dorothea Trudel as well other European faith homes in the summer of 1873. At the conclusion of this four-month pilgrimage, Boardman did not return to America with Cullis. Instead, he went to England and remained there until 1875 helping to establish, with the husband-wife team of Robert Pearsall Smith (1827–1899) and Hannah Whitall Smith (1832–1911), the Higher Life Movement in Europe.[33] Although Boardman became convinced of the verity of faith healing as a result of his European tour, he was reluctant to promote it. By 1880, however, Boardman publicly proclaimed his belief in faith healing and began a healing ministry in Sweden. He also began writing a book on divine healing that would become Cullis's "standard apologetic" for the doctrine of faith healing. That book, *The Great Physician (Jehovah Rophi)*, was published by Cullis's Repository.[34]

In 1882 Boardman opened a faith healing home, Bethshan, in London.[35] The use of medicine or physicians was not allowed. In 1885, Boardman convened the first international faith healing conference in London, the International Conference on Divine Healing and Holiness. Boardman achieved what earlier leaders of the movement, including Cullis, had not achieved, namely, a theological defense of divine healing.

In 1881 A. B. Simpson (1843–1919), in failing health, attended Cullis's faith convention and became convinced of Christ's healing power through Cullis's preaching, through testimonies of people who had been healed, and through biblical revelation. As a result, Simpson wrote a three-part pledge declaring his commitment to the doctrine of divine healing. After making this pledge and experiencing "tingling with a sense of God's presence" in his body, Simpson declared himself healed. He resigned as pastor of the Thirteenth Street Presbyterian Church in New York City and founded an independent church, Gospel Tabernacle, a place where all people, especially the poor, were welcome. He began his independent ministry hoping that it would enable him to fulfill his vision of evangelizing the "unchurched masses." Along with Gospel Tabernacle, Simpson founded the Missionary Union for the Evangelization of the World in 1883. This organization became the Evangelical Missionary Alliance in 1887, the same year that he founded the Christian Alliance. In 1897 both groups combined to form a new denomination, the Christian and Missionary Alliance, based on Simpson's "Fourfold Gospel: Christ our Savior, Sanctifier, Healer and Coming King."[36]

Most important, Simpson considered divine healing the most effective feature of his ministry. He conducted Friday afternoon healing meetings in Gospel Tabernacle for thirty-eight years. These renowned healing services were attended by thousands from New York City and from around the country. Besides testi-

monies of healing, Bible teaching on healing, and praying for
and anointing the sick with oil, Simpson's Friday meetings included prayer for thousands who had written to Simpson requesting prayer for healing. Simpson also founded a faith home
for prayer and healing. Modeled on Cullis's faith home, Berachah Home, like the Friday healing meetings, created such interest that several faith homes were established over the next
few years that were directly or indirectly connected to Simpson's ministry. Another vital component of Simpson's healing
ministry was the annual faith convention he held at Old Orchard
Beach, beginning in the summer of 1886. Convened around the
theme "Christian Life and Work and Divine Healing," Simpson's
ten-day conventions endured for thirty-two years and extended
the faith convention as an institution for twenty years after
Cullis's death. Simpson's conventions demonstrated even further the alliance between the Holiness and faith healing movements. Prominent evangelicals who were active in both the
Holiness and faith healing movements, including D. L. Moody,
Phoebe Palmer, Carrie Judd, A. J. Gordon, Otto Stockmayer, and
Mrs. Michael Baxter, spoke at these conventions.[37]

Simpson also published healing testimonies in his magazine,
Word, Work, and World, and wrote several books about divine
healing, including *The Gospel of Healing.* Simpson did not con-
done the use of medicine or physicians as he believed both reflected doubt about the reality of divine healing.[38] By continuing
the work begun by Charles Cullis, he helped ensure the
longevity and growth of the divine healing movement into the
twentieth century.

A. J. Gordon (1836–1895), a trustee of Cullis's Faith Work,
was another important figure in the divine healing movement.
Gordon, pastor of the Clarendon Street Baptist Church in
Boston, was a major apologist for the doctrine of faith healing,
and his writings constitute a major contribution to the faith

healing movement. In addition to founding a periodical, *The Watchword*, in 1878, Gordon wrote several books, including *The Ministry of Healing: Miracles of Cure in All Ages.*[39]

Faith Healing Defended

The doctrine of faith healing provoked controversy and debate among theologians, clergy, and religious press editors. The controversy centered on interpretation of scriptural passages related to healing and on whether miraculous cures could still appear or whether they had ended with the apostolic age. One of the most vehement critics of the faith cure movement was James Buckley (1836–1920), editor of the Methodist *Christian Advocate*, a position he held from 1880 to 1912. Chappell argues that the *Christian Advocate* "moved steadily from a position of cautious neutrality to one of open hostility under the leadership of Buckley."[40] In *Faith-Healing, Christian Science and Kindred Phenomena*, Buckley argued the "harmful effects" of believing in faith healing:

> It sets up false grounds for determining whether a person is or is not in the favor of God. It opens the door to every superstition, such as attaching importance to dreams; signs; opening the Bible at random . . . Practically it gives support to other delusions which claim a supernatural element. It seriously diminishes the influence of Christianity by subjecting it to a test which it cannot endure . . . Little hope exists of freeing those already entangled, but it is highly important to prevent others from falling into so plausible and luxurious a snare, and to show that Christianity is not to be held responsible for aberrations of the imagination.[41]

In their theological and doctrinal writings, Boardman, Simpson, and Gordon not only defended faith healing against the attacks of Buckley and other critics, they also developed a systematic theological and biblical framework in which to understand both the practice and doctrine of faith healing. Besides responding to the issue of miraculous cures, they also theorized about the Atonement, specifically about healing as a part of Christ's atoning sacrifice.[42]

In *The Great Physician* Boardman presented Christ not only as a pardoning Savior, but also as a deliverer of sin's consequences, including disease.[43] By examining biblical accounts of healing in both the Hebrew Bible and the New Testament, Boardman argued that "healing was an integral part of the daily work of the primitive Church, and that the Epistle of James unquestionably made healing a permanent provision of the Church's ministry for all eras."[44]

Simpson's theological and doctrinal positions on divine healing, revealed especially in *The Gospel of Healing*, reflected the "normative" views of the faith healing movement. For example, Simpson agreed that illness occurred because of the Fall of Adam and Eve. He believed that Christ, the atoning sacrifice, was the basic principle of divine healing and that atonement included redemption of the body. Similarly, in *The Ministry of Healing: Miracles of Cure in All Ages* and other writings, Gordon argued that Christ's twofold earthly ministry involved healing the sick and forgiving the sinner. Like Simpson, he argued that the Atonement of Christ included bodily healing and that "Christ was both the sickness-bearer and the sin-bearer of his people."[45] Gordon also stated that the conditions for miracles were "the power of Christ and the faith of men" and that with the manifestation of a "revival of primitive faith and apostolic simplicity there we find a profession of the chaste and evangelical miracles which characterized the apostolic age."[46] Gordon's *The Ministry of Healing*, which earned respect from the critics of faith healing, is today regarded as an important theological statement on faith healing.[47] While this group of Cullis's disciples may have differed over the use of medicine in faith healing, their theological contribution had a major impact on the movement.[48]

Additionally, although Cullis, Boardman, Simpson, and Gordon were influential in institutionalizing and legitimizing faith healing in the 1880s, Ethan O. Allen, although aged, was still active as a healing evangelist and was recognized for his ministry by Cullis and Simpson. Allen participated in Cullis's faith conventions. And Cullis published Allen's book about his experiences, *Faith Healing: or What I Have Witnessed of the Fulfillment of James V: 14, 15, 16*. Recognizing Allen's pioneering faith healing ministry, Simpson called him the "Father of Divine Healing."[49]

Women and Healing

In the 1880s faith healing began to receive more publicity, numerous healing conventions were held, faith cure homes were established, and a variety of periodicals and popular testimonial works were published. Most important, during this formative period of the divine healing movement, women occupied a central role as practitioners, matrons, and operators of faith homes. Some matrons had received healing at Cullis's faith conventions or in his Boston faith home, established in 1882, which, along with the faith homes established by Dorothea Trudel in Switzerland, was the model for the numerous faith homes established by women in the early 1880s.[50]

Although faith homes differed slightly in terms of how they were run and the accommodations offered, all shared a basic purpose: to pray for the sick individually and to instruct them in the biblical teaching on faith healing. Faith homes also provided comfort and rest for the sick as their journey toward full restoration of health continued. The length of stay generally ranged from a few days to four weeks. When she began Faith-Rest Cottage, in 1882, Carrie Judd wrote that her faith home was not a "permanent" home. Judd described the purpose of her home as follows: "It has been instituted for the accommodation of those out of the city who wish to come here and attend our faith-meeting, and who desire to meet others of like precious faith for their mutual strengthening in the Lord."[51] The time spent at a faith home was often determined by its size. At the larger, more popular homes, such as Simpson's Berachah Home and Carrie Judd's Faith-Rest Cottage, the large number of requests determined who could be accommodated and for how long. No fee was charged at faith homes. Simpson and Judd publicized their faith homes through their publications and received support, both financial and material, for this aspect of their ministries. Carrie Judd relates receiving "a beautiful silver caster, butter dish and knife," from Anna Prosser's Bible class.[52] By 1887 more than thirty faith homes, many of them operated by women, existed.[53]

Women also had prominent roles as speakers at faith conventions and as writers of some of the most important healing testimonial and general works on the theology of faith healing. Women also founded and edited journals devoted exclusively to faith healing and to faith healing and Holiness. In 1881 Carrie Judd began publishing her journal devoted to faith healing and Holiness, *Triumphs of Faith*.[54] "Judd," according to Paul Chappell, "made a distinctive contribution in her publication by identifying healing ministries conducted by females and including articles by dozens of women who ministered in the movement." He lists, along with Sarah Mix, the names of twenty-nine women, including a physician.[55] Sarah Mix also began publishing her journal *Victory Through Faith*.

Some journals, compilations of healing testimonials, and general works on faith healing were published on both sides of the Atlantic and in several editions. For example, Mrs. Michael Baxter, a leader in the faith healing movement in England, founded a periodical, *The Healer*, which was read by adherents and practitioners of faith healing in the United States as well as in England. Baxter also regularly contributed articles to journals published in the United States, including Cullis's *Times of Refreshing* and Judd's *Triumphs of Faith*.[56] With Mrs. Baxter's help, Carrie Judd's *The Prayer of Faith*, first published in 1880, was reprinted four times and published in German, French, Swedish, and Dutch, thus giving her international attention and, by extension, also giving international attention to Sarah Mix, whose prayers had led to Judd's healing.[57]

Both Ethan O. Allen and Charles Cullis encouraged women as full and equal participants in the faith healing movement. Because the Holiness movement was open to and encouraged women's leadership, and because of the exemplary ministry of Phoebe Palmer, it is not unusual that Allen would choose Sarah Mix and other women as collaborators in his ministry. In addition to engaging women as assistants, Allen supported women who were beginning ministries in faith healing, mainly as founders and operators of faith homes and as healing evangelists. For example, Allen assisted Mary Shoemaker, one of his later assistants, in establishing Shiloh Chapel, a faith home in Springfield, Massachusetts.[58] Allen also included visits to faith homes in his ministry itinerary. One of these was the Four-fold Gospel Mission in Troy, New York, established by Sara Musgrove, another woman Allen supported. Musgrove, who found healing through Allen's healing ministry, maintained her faith

home for forty-one years. In Buffalo, New York, Allen visited
Carrie Judd's Faith-Rest Cottage.[59] Both Musgrove and Judd became prominent in Simpson's Christian and Missionary Alliance,
one of the new denominations established during this period
that included faith healing as one of its basic doctrines. Cullis
also included Sarah Mix, Carrie Judd, Mrs. Phoebe Upham, and
Hannah Whitall Smith, leaders in the Holiness movement, as regular speakers at his faith conventions.[60] Despite James Buckley's
vehement opposition to the movement, he recognized Sarah Mix
as "the instrument of the cure of persons who have devoted
themselves to faith-healing, attending conventions, writing
books, etc. Her death was bewailed by many respectable persons, without distinction of creed, sex, age, or color, who believed that they had been cured through her prayers." [61]

Faith Healing as Religious Experience

It is difficult to know with certainty how many evangelicals believed in the doctrine of faith healing, attended faith conventions, and subscribed to various periodicals devoted to faith
healing or to faith healing and Holiness. In his study of the faith
cure movement, Raymond Cunningham argues that most evangelicals who embraced perfection did not embrace faith healing.
Historical evidence points to the fact that, as with the Holiness
movement, there was a movement of "come-outism" within the
divine healing movement. As indicated earlier, A. B. Simpson
and other preachers who were advocates and practitioners of
faith healing renounced their denominational affiliations and
formed independent ministries. According to Chappell, "By so
doing, these men created extensive and permanent structures
by which to perpetuate the message of divine healing world-
wide." Also, countless individuals left denominations for inde-

pendent churches "where the supernatural workings of God were evident."[62] Conversely, denominational loyalists were less likely to preach healing.

Cunningham further argues that religious belief did not necessarily evoke interest in faith healing. Interest in faith healing, he states, must be viewed alongside the rise of "mind cure" during this period. Cunningham observes:

> The theoretical foundations of "faith cure" and "mind cure" were totally different, but the common element was the hope both offered of relief from many symptoms which regular medical practice seemed unable to treat effectively. . . . From the vantage point of later developments in both religion and medicine, perhaps the principal significance of the faith cure movement was that it publicized, for the first time, a concept of salvation that included health as an integral part of it.[63]

Cunningham's assertion that faith cure and mind cure offered hope to countless individuals whose suffering was not alleviated by nineteenth-century medicine is documented in the historical record. His argument that the "theoretical foundations" of both approaches to healing were "totally different," however, is subject to qualification and calls for reassessment. Advocates and practitioners in both movements emphasized and were concerned with religious experience and an experience of the supernatural. Although it is important to acknowledge the distinctiveness of faith cure and mind cure, our understanding of both movements is enriched by seeing their similarities. Mary Baker Eddy and Christian Science, the movement she founded, provide historical evidence to qualify Cunningham's argument. Christian Science teaching and Eddy's religious experience show the commonality of Christian theology, the centrality of the person of Christ, and a belief in spiritual power to heal in both faith cure and mind cure.[64]

First, Mary Baker Eddy (1821–1910), like Sarah Mix, experienced the healing power of Jesus.[65] In 1866 in Lynn, Massachusetts, Eddy fell on an icy sidewalk and suffered serious injury which left her a semi-invalid. She recounts praying and reading a New Testament passage detailing one of Jesus' healings and, as a result, claimed healing. Robert Peel describes her healing as follows: "The words of Jesus flooded into her thought, 'I am the way, the truth, and the life: no man cometh unto the Father but by me,' and quite suddenly she was filled with the conviction that her life was in God—that God was the only Life, the only I AM. At that moment she was healed."[66] Eddy's realization underscores the emphasis on Jesus as healer, a belief that was central to both faith cure and Christian Science. At the same time, it points to an important difference, namely Eddy's vision in which "she saw all being as spiritual, divine, immortal, wholly good. There was no room for fear or pain or death, no room for the limits that men define as matter."[67] The salvific role of Jesus, moreover, was not paramount; rather, in Christian Science, Jesus' healing powers could be acquired by others.

Second, Mary Baker Eddy considered Christian Science "Christian." She defended her movement and theology before a gathering of nearly three thousand in Tremont Temple in Boston on March 16, 1885.[68] The impetus for this address was the criticism of Christian Science by A. J. Gordon, who, as mentioned earlier, was an important apologist for the doctrine of faith healing. In a letter Gordon wrote to Reverend Joseph Cook (1838–1901), a Congregationalist and convenor of a weekly gathering, the Monday Lectures, Gordon argued that Christian Science denied the Atonement, a central tenet of Christianity, and the personality of God. Eddy responded to Gordon (and Cook) on these points as follows:

Do I believe in a personal God?

I believe in God as the Supreme Being. I know not what
the person of omnipotence and omnipresence is, or what
the infinite includes; therefore, I worship that of which I
can conceive, first, as a loving Father and Mother; then, as
thought ascends the scale of being to diviner consciousness, God becomes to me, as to the apostle who declared
it, "God is Love,"—divine Principle,—which I worship;
and "after the manner of my fathers, so worship I God."

Do I believe in the atonement of Christ?

I do; and this becomes more to me since it includes
man's redemption from sickness as well as from sin. I rev-
erence and adore Christ as never before.

It brings to my sense, and to the sense of all who enter-
tain this understanding of the Science of God, a *whole* salvation.[69]

This view of the Atonement was consonant with the "normative"
view of the Atonement in the divine healing movement, even as
espoused by A. B. Simpson and A. J. Gordon.

Third, both movements emphasized the sick person's frame
of mind at the time of healing. According to faith cure practitioners, one had to demonstrate faith and belief in God's promise to heal or, in the words of Sarah Mix, to "act faith." Believing
the biblical promise in the Epistle of James, faith healing practitioners prayed, laid hands on the sick, and (some practitioners)
anointed the sick person with oil. Conversely, in Christian Science, the knowledge of the unreality and illusiveness of matter,
including sin, evil, sickness, and suffering, was the requisite
frame of mind for receiving Christian Science treatment. As
Stephen Gottschalk points out, for Eddy, "her Christian Science
treatment was truly prayer."[70] As she wrote in *Science and
Health:* "The prayer that reforms the sinner and heals the sick is

an absolute faith that all things are possible to God,—a spiritual understanding of Him, an unselfed love."[71] It was common for healing practitioners in both movements to help others find healing over distance. One did not need to be in the physical presence of a healing practitioner to receive the prayer of faith, as was certainly the case in the ministry of Sarah Mix. In fact, it was standard practice among faith healing practitioners to offer the healing prayer of faith through correspondence. In Christian Science, this practice was called "absent treatment."

Eddy explained, "Christian Science recognizing the capabilities of Mind to act of itself, and independent of matter, enables one to heal cases without even having seen the individual,—or simply after having been made acquainted with the mental condition of the patient."[72] Christian Scientists' basis for this practice was the biblical example of Jesus' healing of the centurion's servant in Matthew 8:5–13. Believing that God's promises to heal were true was important for evangelicals who sought bodily healing from the ministry of a faith healing practitioner.

Both movements differed internally and externally over the use of medicine and physicians while seeking healing from a practitioner. Sarah Mix and other healing practitioners in the 1880s discouraged the use of medicine and physicians as indicating a sick person's lack of faith. On the other hand, Christian Science argued extensively over the use of medicine and physicians. Eddy's establishment of her Metaphysical College was one way of dealing with this belief.

Finally, in both movements testimony was important. As mentioned earlier, personal testimony attesting to God's promise to heal was an important element in the faith healing movement. Personal testimony encouraged others to believe the biblical promises of healing and helped to disseminate the doctrine of faith healing. In the same manner, in Christian Science "demonstration" reflected the importance of testimony, or provability of the true nature of reality and of God. Demonstration, Eddy believed, would convince others of the veracity of her teaching on healing. In the Christian Science *Manual*, Eddy wrote: "Testimony in regard to healing of the sick is highly important. More than a mere rehearsal of blessings, it scales the pinnacles of praise and illustrates the demonstration of Christ."[73]

Cunningham's argument that the theoretical foundations of both approaches to healing were totally different also needs to be reassessed in light of the argument Chappell presents in the conclusion to his study of the divine healing movement. Although he does not indicate that his conclusion is a refutation of Cunningham's statement, Chappell does, in fact, posit a different view. He argues that adherents of faith healing were motivated by a desire "to see and experience God in living commerce with His creation."[74] The early leaders of the movement were lay people, which gave the movement a "grassroots" character, and Chappell further argues that the "common people" desired to see God "demonstrate once again His reality in human affairs through the supernatural. These people stressed the pragmatic aspects of God's dealing with His people and were results oriented. Thus, they placed strong stress upon the experiential and gave prominence to personal testimonies as a way of sharing the truth of divine healing."[75]

Additionally, we can reexamine Cunningham's argument in light of recent scholarship on various aspects of mind cure. Most notably, Ann Taves's recent study helps us to understand both faith cure and mind cure from the perspective of religious experience. Her study supports and expands the ideas Chappell discussed in his conclusion. As Taves's study demonstrates, Protestant evangelical religion was the common theoretical foundation for both faith cure and mind cure. Such mental therapies as mesmerism emerged from the nineteenth-century emphasis on religious experience. Whereas Wesleyan Holiness emphasized an experience of the supernatural through sanctification, mind cure also emphasized the experience of the supernatural through such phenomena as mesmeric trance, dreams, and visions. Cunningham failed to see that the difference between mind cure and faith cure had more to do with explanations of these religious experiences than with "theoretical foundations." Taves argues the importance of "recontextualizing explanations of experience in their own traditions of discourse and practice."[76]

Faith cure and mind cure thus had in common the beliefs of nineteenth-century evangelical Protestantism and a strong belief in the spiritual power of healing. Yet, despite this common ground, as I have indicated in my examination of the divine healing movement, there were also significant differences between these two healing movements.

The nineteenth-century divine healing movement had an enormous impact on the religious experience of evangelical Protestants. The legacy of that movement has continued into the twentieth and twenty-first centuries in Pentecostalism and in charismatic traditions that emphasize healing by faith and the laying on of hands. The faith healing evangelists of the nineteenth century were first and foremost women and men of prayer whose prayers were offered for the bodily healing of the sick. Additionally, they taught others the biblical meaning of healing. For many faith healing practitioners, healing of the body and the soul went together. As journalist Frank Townsend observed:

> Some things about this recent movement distinguish it from any previous modern miracles. . . . The asserted cures are not used for the aggrandizement of any special denomination or religious system. They are performed

gratuitously. Those who work them claim no unusual powers, saying that such deeds may be done by any Christian
of enough faith. They give all the glory to God, to whose
power they ascribe the miracles. And they seem to be,
without exception, persons whose lives are pure and
whose motives are above suspicion.[77]

This approach to healing changes in the early twentieth century
with the rise of Pentecostalism and a movement away from the
practice of the prayer of faith to healing through the laying on of
hands.

Sarah Mix: Faith Healing, African American Healing Traditions, and African American Women's Healing Work

As a faith healing evangelist, Sarah Mix reflects an historical
continuum of healing that includes not only faith healing but,
equally important, a complex and multifaceted African American healing tradition that dates from Africa and continues to
this day. As historian Albert Raboteau has noted, blacks' views
about healing, medicine, and religion have their roots in Africa.
These beliefs and their accompanying practices were imported
to the American colonies during the Atlantic slave trade and
continued even as blacks adopted and assimilated Christianity
and other religious traditions. Herbalism, astrology, and conjure, for example, flourished in the slave quarters and were
viewed not only as being compatible with Christianity, but also
as complementing it.[78]

According to Raboteau, conjure, also known as "voodoo" and
"rootworking," among other names, provided explanations for
illness, suffering, and other human experiences that Protestantism failed to address until the advent of the Holiness and

Pentecostal movements. Both movements emphasized the gifts of the Holy Spirit, including the gift of healing.[79] Raboteau's argument, I believe, helps to show the connection between an African American healing tradition that includes faith healing, or, more accurately, faith *and* healing. In both faith healing and African American healing traditions, those seeking healing were concerned with results and desired to see a demonstration of supernatural power in the affairs of their daily lives. Furthermore, the approach to healing found in conjure (and in conjure coupled with Christianity) may also help to explain why the faith healing movement, more than various mind cures such as Christian Science, would appeal to Sarah Mix and other African Americans in the nineteenth century.

African Americans connected faith and healing, whether or not they were actively involved in the faith healing movement as practitioners or were ministered to by a faith healing evangelist. Sharla Fett points out this connection in the conversion narrative of a former slave woman that included an account of her healing from swollen limbs by "Doctor Jesus." She prays, asking God to relieve her misery, and testifies:

> The spirit directed me to get some peach-tree leaves and beat them up and put them about my limbs. I did this, and in a day or two that swelling left me, and I haven't been bothered since. More than this, I don't remember ever paying out but three dollars for doctor's bills in my life either for myself, my children, or my grandchildren. Doctor Jesus tells me what to do.[80]

In a similar manner, well-known Holiness evangelist Amanda Berry Smith recounts in her autobiography that she ceased to use medicine for nearly two years, although suffering pains in her neck and back. She says, "The Lord was my physician."[81]

When she becomes ill with a severe cold, she indicates that God instructs her to use a simple, unspecified remedy to alleviate her suffering. Although Smith relates her experience within a larger discussion on divine healing, her story demonstrates a broader meaning of faith healing, or faith and healing, especially for African Americans.

Sarah Mix also reflects an historical continuum of African American female healing practitioners. In her examination of black women's healing work, especially herbalism and bedside care, Sharla Fett points out that during slavery black women performed a variety of healing roles, including "hospital nurse," "midwife," and "doctoress."[82] These roles were performed within the plantation community, for slaveholders and slaves alike. Whether routine everyday tasks such as nursing and treating injuries, or "doctoring," or conjuration, all relied on spiritual empowerment for effectiveness, and all forms of healing were expressions of religious belief. According to Fett, "Many women healers, as well as some men, spoke in an explicitly Christian language of God working through them."[83]

This tradition of African American healing women paved the way for Mix's successful ministry with the sick, especially whites. Recognizing Mix's effectiveness and spiritual power to facilitate healing, whites apparently sought her out for healing through prayer and the laying on of hands. Because Europeans, like Africans, brought to the American colonies a system of magic, lore, and wonders and had in common with African Americans many supernatural beliefs and practices,[84] it therefore would have been easy for both blacks and whites, accustomed to seeking out black healing practitioners of all sorts, to seek out Sarah Mix for healing through prayer. Additionally, there could have been a carryover from slavery in that blacks and whites saw Sarah Mix's ministry, like domestic work, as a service to render. Blacks and whites relied on slave women's skills as healers. As Fett observes with respect to the relationship between healing and female domestic labor during slavery,

> Nursing and midwifery involved a panoply of domestic skills, since slave healers did not merely keep watch over the sick and women in labor. They made medicines, prepared food, and washed the bodies and bedclothes of the sick. Healing work thus overlapped with domestic tasks of cooking, cleaning, and laundering. The close association between healing and female domestic labor imbued healing with elements of skill and servitude.[85]

Perhaps Mix, like her formerly enslaved sisters, was viewed by some as performing a service in her faith healing ministry, especially as an operator of a faith home. Although we lack specific details about how Mix operated her faith home in her Torrington residence, we can assume that she performed some domestic tasks even as she carried on her ministry of teaching faith healing and praying for those who came for healing.

Sarah Mix's healing ministry might also be looked at metaphorically. In addition to addressing physical pain and suffering in her healing ministry, she also may have addressed divisions between blacks and whites indirectly. Although not explicitly stated in her spiritual autobiography or in other writings, or alluded to in the testimonials she compiled, one is led to wonder if the healing of the cultural wounds of racial oppression and gender discrimination may have underlain Mix's vision of healing and wholeness. As Raboteau has pointed out, "Sacred medicines, according to African belief, were given by God not only to protect individual well-being, but also to insure societal well-being. They were meant to heal the body social as well as the body personal."[86] Mix, empowered by the Holy Spirit and a deep religious faith, could also have been motivated by this

African belief as she helped others find healing and relief from their physical suffering and pain. The "sacred medicine" she offered was the prayer of faith and the laying on of hands. Mix offered hope and healing to blacks and whites, to sick individuals and others needing healing of body and soul. In the words of the Negro spiritual, Sarah Mix was "a balm in Gilead, to make the wounded whole."

"Go Work in My Vineyard": Biographical Sketch of Sarah Mix

Sarah Ann Freeman Mix was born May 5, 1832, in Torrington, Litchfield County, Connecticut, to Datus and Lois Freeman. She grew up in a family of thirteen. Her parents, although free, endured financial hardship and sent Mix out to work in domestic service after she had acquired a rudimentary education. Although her parents were "professing Christians" (see p. 201) when they married, her father, she writes, came to "neglect the family altar" (p. 201). Her mother, a member of the Baptist church in Newfield, Connecticut, "overwhelmed with cares, trials, and perplexities gave up to all human appearance" (p. 201). Despite her parents' lack of consistent religious faith, Mix did attend Sabbath School. Her desire to be a Christian was prompted by stories of conversion she read in Sabbath School books. As is typical of spiritual autobiographies, Mix minimizes details about her family, childhood, and youth, and emphasizes the process of her religious conversion. The conversion process, which could last for years, included certain essential steps. A keen awareness of one's sinfulness and resulting separation from God was an essential first step toward salvation.[87]

Sarah Mix first identified what she deemed her sinful nature when she was a seven-year-old girl. She writes: "I felt I was so wicked I could go silently out into the garden and hide myself in the pea vines, and there kneel in my childlike manner and ask God to make me a better child" (p. 201). When her brother dies when less than four years old, Mix is again convinced that she is "so wicked" (p. 202). Her conviction, however, does not lead to conversion. Rather, Mix seeks "pleasure and comfort in sin and folly" (p. 202). In his discussion of the spiritual autobiographies of Jarena Lee, Julia Foote, and Zilpha Elaw, three nineteenth-century black women preachers, William Andrews notes a similar depiction of childhood: "Each woman extracts from her childhood instances of thoughtlessness, frivolity, or willfulness, which are highlighted to signify an early state of spiritual lostness and hopelessness." This portrayal of childhood is rather typical of American spiritual autobiography.[88]

After her father's death from consumption, Mix and her mother move to New Haven, and Mix assumes primary responsibility for their basic needs by working as a domestic. Suffering poverty and illness, Mix continues striving with God. Her intense spiritual struggle, characterized by equally intense resistance, continued into early adulthood. Between the time of their arrival in New Haven and her mother's death almost three years later, Mix is converted when "a great outpouring of the spirit of God" (p. 203) occurs in New Haven churches. She attended a three-week revival at Bethel AME (African Methodist Episcopal) Church and struggled not only with yielding to God, but also with the emotionalism of the revival itself. "But, the burden became so heavy," she explains, "it seemed as if I must die and be lost at last. I finally said any way, 'Oh Lord save me from destruction'" (p. 204). The night of her conversion Mix approaches the altar resolved not to make any "loud noise or groan" (p. 204), is overcome with emotion, and is unable to refrain from expressing her deepest feelings. In the most compelling and dramatic section of her spiritual autobiography, Mix describes her conversion as follows:

My agonies were indescribable. I began to beg and cry aloud for mercy. The last I remembered of myself in that condition I was crying at the top of my voice, "Lord, save or I perish." I was then lost to all around me, and the first recollection of anything was seemingly a white cloud coming from God out of heaven. It came nearer and nearer until I was engulfed in it. Sin was washed away, the burden of guilt was removed and I could say, "Come all the world, and I will tell you what the Lord has done for me." I shouted and praised God until I lost my strength and was obliged to be led home. I shouted "Glory to God" all the way through the streets. (p. 204)

Following her conversion Mix and her mother, who has rededicated herself to God, continue contending with poverty but are sustained by their belief that God will provide for them. Mix's mother dies, and in 1855 Mix herself becomes ill with consumption and is not expected to live. Her physician suggests that Mix, who was now living in New York City, leave the city and prescribes "tincture of barks . . . dieting and . . . fresh air" (p. 207). Mix recuperates at her sister's home in Goshen, Connecticut, and is well enough in two months to resume work as a domestic. The following spring, at the age of twenty-three, she marries Edward M. Mix, on March 9, 1856.

Sarah Mix reveals that since the death of her mother she had become "indifferent and cold spiritually" (p. 207) and her husband had also "wandered from God" (p. 207). The Mixes renewed their faith and became Adventists.[89] Their faith, however, was severely tested as, one by one, all seven of their children died at an early age. As Sarah Mix reflects on the loss of her children, she comes to believe that God is calling her "to do something more for him than I had ever done" (p. 207). At the time

Mix was a dressmaker. She relates that she hears a voice saying "Go work to-day in my vineyard" (p. 208).

Mix prays, asking God for a sign that he has indeed spoken to her and called her to ministry. She relates two visionary dreams that affirm God's call and cause Mix to believe God's message to her. This part of Mix's narrative is also congruent with the pattern of American spiritual autobiography and visionary experience, especially in African American spiritual autobiography. We are reminded on the one hand of Jarena Lee and on the other of Shaker visionary and preacher Rebecca Cox Jackson, whose remarkable spiritual autobiography records her dreams and visions.[90] Andrews observes that visionary experiences were particularly important for women, "for through these visionary moments they saw themselves transformed, inspirited, and, for the first time, chosen for a providential purpose."[91] Such was certainly the case with Sarah Mix, who yields to God's call to "Go work to-day in my vineyard" (p. 208). While she writes that "The Lord . . . has blessed the labors" (p. 210), Mix does not provide details about the type of ministry she has. She only mentions not feeling well when she has gone to "fill an appointment" (p. 210). We can infer from this statement that she is referring to her healing ministry.

The remainder of Mix's narrative briefly mentions her healing through the healing ministry of Ethan O. Allen on December 19, 1877, her "gift of healing," and the opposition to her faith healing ministry.[92] Criticism and opposition, however, do not deter Mix. She affirms her faith in God and her commitment to obey God's call to her. She writes: "I had rather wear out in the vineyard of my Master than to rust out in idleness" (p. 210).

In an appendix to *The Life*, Edward Mix writes about his wife's failing health, her last days, and her death. Although she had claimed healing of consumption, as noted earlier, on December 19, 1877, when Allen laid hands on her, the disease recurred about four years later. Edward Mix prayed for his wife and laid hands on her. Allen also prayed a second time for Sarah Mix's healing from consumption, and an unnamed healer also prayed and laid hands on Mix. These prayers, however, did not effect a long-term cure. What is interesting in this appendix is Edward Mix's discussion about doubt, especially as it relates to his wife's healing. Although Mix herself stressed the importance of faith, Edward Mix, it seems, seeks to assert that his wife was not healed because of doubt. Why did Edward Mix question his wife's faith? Although Sarah and Edward Mix ministered together, Sarah was the better known of the two.[93] In view of his wife's popularity and highly-esteemed reputation as a faith healing practitioner, one wonders if Edward Mix felt he could now have a career on his own. Was he trying to discredit Mix or undermine her ministry in order to make a name for himself? Or was he simply using this opportunity to exhort others about the role of faith in healing? Is he offering an apologetic for the doctrine of faith healing, specifically his wife's ministry in light of opposition to her as a faith healing evangelist? Given the information available, it is not possible to answer these questions definitively. We do know that Edward Mix moved to Newport, Rhode Island, and became an Elder in the Shiloh Baptist Church. In a history of the church published in 1901, he is described as "being actively engaged in the service of his Master."[94]

Despite Edward Mix's exhortation on the necessity of faith in healing, especially with respect to his wife, he does acknowledge her successful ministry. He points out that, even as her health deteriorated, Mix continued preaching and offering prayers for healing, often traveling hundreds of miles and preaching nightly until very late. He writes: "She seemed to be moved by an unseen power. If she could write to some sick one, or pray for them, then she was happy" (p. 215). Sarah Mix also continued her weekly

Wednesday prayer time even after the women who had regularly attended Mix's prayer meeting eventually lost interest and stopped attending. Often, Mix prayed alone. Edward Mix offers to send to readers a photograph of his wife for twenty-five cents and one of them together for fifty cents. He promises to continue the prayer meeting for the sick and also promotes *Faith Cures, and Answers to Prayer*, which he describes as "a great help to them that are learning the way of faith."[95]

Sarah Mix died April 14, 1884, at the age of fifty-one, from consumption. She believed that she had been faithful to God's calling: "I do believe there is a crown laid up for me; and there will be some stars to deck my crown with in the day of Christ's coming." Believing that her words would inspire those who would read of her life, she prayed at the end of her spiritual autobiography: "May the blessing of God rest upon all who shall read of my imperfect life, is the prayer of unworthy me. Amen" (p. 211)

As a text written by a black woman in the nineteenth century, *The Life of Mrs. Edward Mix, Written By Herself* belongs not only to the black American literary tradition. It also exemplifies the traditions of American spiritual autobiography and black women's spiritual narratives. It is very similar in form and content to *The Life and Religious Experience of Jarena Lee, A Coloured Lady*, published in 1836.[96] For the modern reader, Mix's spiritual autobiography raises many questions. Because of the striking similarity between *The Life* and Jarena Lee's autobiography, one wonders if Mix's text was deliberately patterned after Lee's. Also, the publication delay leads one to ask if Mix had planned to write a longer spiritual autobiography that would include more information about her faith healing ministry. Or did Mix deliberately end her narrative with only a brief mention of her activities as a healing evangelist because of the opposition she faced in her ministry?

The fact that Mix wrote a spiritual autobiography attests to her literacy and education as well as to the importance she attached to her life as a public figure. Although Paul Chappell describes Mix as a "well educated, articulate, and persuasive person," there is no evidence supporting Mix's acquiring of more than a rudimentary education.[97] Mix describes herself as "illiterate" and having "no talent" (p. 208), but this was more a statement of humility and reliance on God's help and inspiration. Possibly Mix was an autodidact. She not only read the Bible and knew how to use a concordance, but was also capable of writing scriptural exegeses on a variety of texts. And, moreover, Mix was an editor, publisher, writer, and lay theologian. Nevertheless, "written by herself" is the way she (like other black writers who did not attach authenticating affidavits by whites to their narratives) authorized her own voice.[98]

"Send for Mrs. Mix and Be Cured"

Faith Cures, and Answers to Prayer, by Mrs. Edward Mix was published in 1882. Believing that her ministry was significant and that God's promises to heal were true, Sarah Mix compiled written testimonials to encourage others to believe the scriptural passages that promised healing, and to make her healing ministry known. Her book was a wellspring of edification, encouragement, and inspiration. Through *Faith Cures*, Mix extended her public ministry as a healing evangelist, teacher and preacher. She also testified. Like the journal she published, *Victory Through Faith*, Mix's book was another way she used the printed word to expand her public ministry and to convey the faith healing doctrine. *Faith Cures* affirms Mix's calling by God to "Go work in my vineyard."

"Does God answer prayer?" This provocative question is the first sentence of the preface to *Faith Cures*. Demonstrating her

biblical understanding of Christian healing as well as her capabilities as both a lay theologian and a preacher, Sarah Mix re-
sponds to this question with scriptural exegeses that emphasize
the importance of faith in healing and her belief that God heals
both body and soul, both physical and spiritual ills (p. 7).[99] Mix,
moreover, believed it was her "duty" to testify to her healing
from consumption and to teach others about faith healing,
specifically that "the prayer of faith shall save the sick" (p. 7).
Mix writes: "Believing as I do, that God's promises are sure, and
that by a blessed and happy experience have proved them as
such, I feel it my duty to lay my experience before the public"
(p. 8). Although Mix refers to her "weakness and insufficiency to
do the work," she goes on to say that she hopes her experience
of healing as well as the testimonies of others will "increase the
faith of some poor suffering ones, who are beyond the reach of
aid from the arm of flesh, and are willing to trust in God for
deliverance" (p. 8).

In the final section of the preface Mix testifies to her own
healing from consumption through the prayers and laying on of
hands by faith-healing pioneer Ethan O. Allen on December 19,
1877. Although Mix also records this event in her autobiography,
in *Faith Cures* she goes into greater detail about her health and
healing and, most importantly, includes an account of Allen's
discernment of her "gift of healing." Contending with a recur-
rence of consumption, Mix informs Allen, who has come to
Goshen, Connecticut, to heal her sister, that her health is poor.
When Allen asks Mix if she believes God will heal her at that moment, she replies affirmatively. Allen and others assembled
in the room pray for her. Mix reports that when Allen laid hands
on her,

    at that moment I believed I was healed . . . and I was so
    overwhelmed with the power of God, I felt that everything

like disease was removed; I felt as light as a feather, as if I could run through a troop, and leap over a wall. I leaped for joy into the other room, shouting victory in the name of Jesus, and I was not afraid to tell it that I was healed of some troubles I had for twenty years, I was relieved of them, praise the name of the Lord. (p. 11)

This healing is followed by an even more unanticipated turn of events, namely Allen's announcement to Mix that he believes she has the "gift of healing." Mix writes she "could hardly believe it to be true" (p. 11) and, as a result, seeks to find out if she does in fact have the gift of healing by using herself as a test case. Noticing a wart under her right eye, she lays her hand on it and prays "in the name of Jesus . . . if I have the gift let this be removed" (p. 12). The wart falls off when she touches it. Mix follows the same pattern of praying and laying her hand upon her body when, a few days later, she becomes ill with diphtheria. She is "cured" within a short time. Both incidents confirmed for Mix her gift of healing. Mix's ministry as a healing evangelist began, therefore, with herself and initially continued among her neighbors in Torrington, Connecticut.[100] As Mix prayed for neighbors, word about her gift of healing through prayer spread. She writes: "I commenced laboring among neighbors. Then the news spread to towns and villages, and cities and states, and I can say, praise the Lord for his goodness and his wonderful works to the children of men" (p. 12).

As a faith healing practitioner, Mix's practice was rooted in "the prayer of faith" in James 5:14–15: "Are any among you sick? They should call for the elders of the church and have them pray over them, anointing them with oil in the name of the Lord. The prayer of faith will save the sick, and the Lord will raise them up; and anyone who has committed sins will be forgiven" (NRSV).

Mix used the same methods as other healers. She anointed the sick individual with oil, laid hands on the person, and prayed for healing. In encouraging the sick to have complete faith and trust in God's power to heal, she advised them not to use medicine.[101] As the testimonials indicate, Mix might visit a sick person more than once, and she was not always present for a healing. In the latter case, Mix established a specific date and time for prayer and wrote letters of encouragement, thus extending her healing ministry through correspondence.

The main section of *Faith Cures*, "Answers to Prayer," includes over seventy testimonials, usually in the form of a letter, from individuals who found healing through Mix. Although these testimonials were requested by Mix, the writers apparently believed that their testimonies would not only witness to Mix's healing ministry but, most importantly, encourage others to believe in God's promises to heal. Although Mix's ministry was evidently concentrated in New England and various northeastern cities in New York and Pennsylvania, this book includes testimonials from individuals living in other regions of the United States and even two letters from England. One of these was written by Joanna Trood Clear at St. Mary's Church, Torquay, Devonshire, England, in 1880, who seemingly had an ongoing correspondence with Mix. The volume also includes newspaper accounts of Mix's healing ministry and testimonials from clergymen and physicians.

In the first section of testimonies, "Victory Through Christ," Sarah Mix establishes her religious authority and her spiritual power as a healing evangelist, and self-consciously affirms her gift of healing through prayer. She also positions herself within the mainstream of the faith cure movement by including letters exchanged between Alice Ball and Carrie Judd as well as Judd's testimony, "Have Faith in God." In addition to Judd, Charles

Cullis and Jennie Smith, known as the "Railroad Evangelist," are also mentioned in testimonies affirming Mix's ministry of healing.[102]

Carrie Judd (1858–1946), perhaps the best known testifier in *Faith Cures*, found healing through the prayers of Sarah Mix in 1879.[103] A white Episcopalian from Buffalo, New York, Judd fell on a stone sidewalk in 1877 and, as a result, incurred a debilitating spinal injury that left her an invalid. All three physicians she sought for medical care were unable to alleviate her suffering. At this time Judd learned of Sarah Mix from a local newspaper. Judd writes:

> I have no doubt that it was ordered by Providence, that, just at this time, there should appear in the daily paper a short account of the wonderful cures performed in answer to the prayers of Mrs. Edward Mix, a colored lady, of Wolcottville, Conn. The article represented her as an earnest, humble Christian, who simply professed to be doing God's work . . . I felt that a letter must be written her in regard to my own case. I had often heard of faith cures before this, and there had been read to me some portions of W. W. Patton's book, "Remarkable Answers to Prayer," but, although not discrediting them, none had ever produced so great an impression on my mind as this short account of Mrs. Mix. I waited a few hours, then requested my sister to write her that I believed her great faith might avail for me, if she would pray for my recovery, even if she were not present to lay her hands upon me. (pp. 37–38)

In her reply to Judd, Mix wrote: "I can encourage you, by the Word of God, that 'according to your faith,' so be it unto you; and besides you have this promise, 'The prayer of faith shall save the sick, and the Lord shall raise him up' " (p. 38). She also assures

Judd that "Whether the person is present or absent, if it is a 'prayer of faith,' it is all the same, and God has promised to raise up the sick ones, and if they have committed sins to forgive them" (p. 38). Mix instructs Judd to begin praying when she receives her letter and sets a specific time for prayer when Mix and her female prayer group in Wolcottville will pray for Judd's healing. Mix further exhorts Judd to "*act faith.*" "It makes no difference how you feel," Mix writes, "but get right out of bed and begin to walk by faith" (p. 39). Judd stops taking medicine and prays with her family at the appointed hour. Able to get up for the first time in two years, Judd considered herself healed and published her testimony in 1880 in *The Prayer of Faith.* [104]

The testimony of Carrie Judd is noteworthy for several reasons. Although Judd was inspired by the Faith Work of Dr. Charles Cullis to "engage in some special work for the Lord," Sarah Mix was a formative influence on Judd. To an extent, Carrie Judd owed her faith healing ministry to Sarah Mix. Judd, in turn, became a model for Maria B. Woodworth-Etter (1844–1924), an itinerant evangelist whose ministry included healing.[105] As Chappell notes about Judd: "As a disciple of Charles Cullis and Mrs. Elizabeth Mix, she multiplied their efforts and touched tens of thousands with the message of healing which they were never to reach." [106] Judd was able to reach thousands largely through her literary work. *The Prayer of Faith* led to requests for prayer and opportunities for speaking. As previously discussed, in 1881 Judd began publishing *Triumphs of Faith* and, in 1882 further extended her healing ministry through her faith healing home, "Faith-Rest Cottage," in Buffalo.

Mix and Judd apparently enjoyed a warm friendship and a collegial relationship as healing evangelists. In her autobiography, *"Under His Wings": The Story of My Life,* Judd writes that after her healing she and Mix exchanged letters on a regular basis, and when Mix, accompanied by her husband, visited Judd in Buffalo she and Mix went to the homes of Judd's sick friends to pray for their healing. Judd describes her affection for Sarah Mix as follows: "I remember so well how glad I was to see her and how I loved her."[107]

In a spirit of mutual support, Sarah Mix and Carrie Judd were spiritual sisters. Judd and Mix both spoke at Cullis's faith conventions. They were also "literary compatriots" as well.[108] Specifically, Judd's public testimony in *The Prayer of Faith* and in various newspapers helped make Sarah Mix and her ministry known to a wider audience. This relationship is also attested to in several testimonials in *Faith Cures*, including those written by Almena J. Cowles, Mrs. Dr. J. A. Bassett, and Mrs. George Guild, all of whom mention first learning of faith healing and Sarah Mix through reading Judd's testimony. Also, most of "Victory Through Christ," which includes letters exchanged between Alice Ball and Carrie Judd, is also chapter 9 in Judd's book *The Prayer of Faith*. The circumstances surrounding the publication of this correspondence are unknown. It is possible that Judd offered this correspondence for Mix to use in her book as another way of supporting Mix and her ministry. Ball's letter includes a reference not only to Judd but to Charles Cullis, an additional affirmation of Mix as a leader in the divine healing movement. Additionally, Mix published at least two articles in Judd's *Triumphs of Faith*: "Holding Fast" and "Have Faith in God."[109]

Both the secular and religious press were interested in the faith cure movement, and various newspapers reported the activities of faith healing practitioners, including Sarah Mix. Accounts of Mix's healing ministry in such newspapers as the *Utica Observer* (New York), the *Danbury News* (Connecticut), and the New Haven *Journal and Courier* (Connecticut) are included in *Faith Cures* and underscore not only the press's interest in the faith cure movement but also its crucial role in disseminating information about various healing practitioners.

Letters addressed "Dear Editor" indicate that newspapers also provided a forum for discussion and debate about the doctrine of faith healing, as demonstrated in a testimony signed "One Who Finds the Promise Sure." The letter, addressed to an un-named newspaper editor, is a response to "A Great Sufferer," who apparently believes that prayer along with skill and experi-ence will result in healing. The writer quotes James 5:15 and goes on to testify to Mix's ministry of healing through prayer:

> Several leading papers . . . have published an account of the marvelous cure of Miss Carrie F. Judd of Buffalo, N.Y., who, it is confidently asserted, was healed in answer to the prayers of a colored woman, Mrs. Mix. I date my own restoration from the hour when I providentially met this same Mrs. Mix. Could I write you a private letter I might refer you to many who have received a like blessing. If you will write to Mrs. Edward Mix, Wolcottville, Conn., you may learn far more than I can tell you (pp. 75–76).

In "Another Instance of Mrs. Mix's Wonderful Instrumentality," in the *Journal and Courier*, Mr. Winans relates the healing of his wife, Mrs. D. C. Winans, through the prayers of Mrs. Mix. Her healing prompts an interesting exchange between unidentified readers of the paper about the theology of faith healing.

Clergymen from the Methodist Episcopal and the Episcopal (Anglican) churches supported Mix and wrote testimonials af-firming Mix's healing ministry and verifying faith cures. For ex-ample, C. F. A. Bielby, rector of St. Mary's-Church-on-the-Hill in Buffalo, New York, wrote to a newspaper editor verifying Carrie Judd's illness and subsequent healing. Similarly, A. H. Mead, pas-tor of the Methodist Episcopal Church in West Haven, Connecti-cut, wrote a letter to the editor of the *Journal and Courier* verifying the illness and faith cure healing of his parishioner, Mrs. Herbert Hall.

Mix's ministry was so successful that physicians referred patients to her.[110] There are testimonials from physicians who wrote in support of the efficacy of Mix's prayers for healing, and the testimony of one physician, Charles Wesley Buvinger, attests to his personal belief in faith healing. (This is probably also the longest testimony, pp. 84–105). Also, some individual testimonies from sick individuals indicate their physicians' positive response to a cure effected by the ministry of Mix. In her account of healing of severe (possibly migraine) headaches, Mrs. Susan Talmage indicates that her physician had recommended that she see Mix. Following her healing, Talmage's physician "was very glad, for he said medicine was doing me no good, and such cases he liked to see the Lord take in hand" (p. 142). When Carrie Wilson's fifteen-year-old daughter is healed of cholera, her physician states that "he could not understand it, but looks upon her case as a miracle" (p. 145).

Besides religious belief, the state of the medical profession made it easier for physicians to accept faith healing. Historian Charles Rosenberg points out that the medical profession had fallen into a state of ill repute between 1830 and 1859, and by 1850 most Americans consulted homeopathic and hydropathic practitioners. Further, because of a lack of uniformity in prescribing drugs, many Americans took responsibility for their own health and well-being by studying health and disease. Clergy demonstrated the most enthusiasm in this self-education effort. "Not only did they continue in some cases, as clergymen and for centuries, to do a bit of their own doctoring, they endorsed patent medicines and supported heterodox medical systems."[111] Given this state of affairs, it is not surprising that physicians and clergy would write healing testimonies and be among the faith cure movement's ardent supporters.

It appears that some individuals went directly to Mix's home for healing rather than first contacting her by letter. This was the case with a Mrs. Lee, who, Mix writes, "came to board with me two weeks" (p. 182). Lee, who had suffered for three years with weak lungs due to back and side pains, was receiving medical care from a physician when she went to stay with Mix. Mix describes Lee's healing as follows:

> I called her down to prayers . . . I prayed for her, and as I prayed, I felt the power of God come upon me. I arose and laid my hands on her in the name of the Lord. The healing power was so strong upon her that she shook and trembled, and lost her strength. . . . She said she felt the power go all through her lungs and down her back; she soon got so she could go upstairs without the least exertion, and could lie on that side as well as ever, and without any of the pains returning. (pp. 182–83)

It was not uncommon for a sick person, after finding healing through Mix, to go to Mix's faith cure home for several days or weeks. This was the case with Mary Mack, who stayed in Mix's home for four weeks, and Mrs. John Chase, who stayed with Mix two weeks and four days. In keeping with the purpose of a "faith cure home," those who went to Mix's Wolcottville residence learned more about faith healing from Mix and usually experienced greater improvement in health. Mrs. George Guild, for example, traveled from Wisconsin to Mix's Connecticut home after experiencing healing as a result of Mix's prayers. Guild spent several days with Mix, "holding sweet communion, with precious seasons of prayer, feeling refreshed and instructed in the company of one whom God has so richly blest to the recovery of so many suffering ones by her prayer of faith" (p. 82). It is clear from these testimonies that as a faith healing practitioner, Mix brought not only bodily healing to the suffering, but spiritual healing as well, and further, she inspired many to have faith and trust in God.

Letters of testimony also open a window onto other aspects of the divine healing movement in the 1880s, especially the struggle to believe and to abandon the use of medicine. Several individuals wrote about their ongoing struggle to, in Mix's words, *"act faith."* This struggle is why testimonies were important. Testimonies were written to encourage belief in God's promises to heal. Also, as these testimonies reveal, it was common to seek out more than one healing practitioner. Often a sick person requesting prayer might experience an immediate physical change, but full recovery and restoration of health was often gradual rather than instantaneous, during which time an individual sought additional prayers of healing from another healing practitioner.

We also learn that Sarah Mix traveled to camp meetings to pray for the sick. How often she did this is difficult to know from the information in her writings. Because of the connection between Holiness and faith healing, many individuals also traveled to Holiness camp meetings to receive prayer for healing. Rose Nettleton mentions seeking out Mix at a camp meeting in Tylerville, Connecticut, in August 1881. "I was quite sure Mrs. Mix would be there; I resolved to see her and be healed . . . On the evening of the 24th I went to the camp ground and found Mrs. Mix's tent" (p. 67). We also learn about other healing practitioners from these testimonies.

Also important in *Faith Cures* are the varied writings by Mix herself, which range from journal entries of healings effected through her prayers to what might be considered Mix's theology of healing. Mix testifies to the efficacy of the prayer of faith in healing and theologizes in such statements as: "God has promised to renew youth and strength if we call upon him for it" (p. 183); "There is no God like our God" (p. 184); and "God always delivers those who trust in Him" (p. 187). Mix also includes an original poem, simply titled, "Composed by Mrs. Mix." The four-stanza poem was written after Mix's prayers restored the voice of Mrs. Royal Cross. Each stanza begins with: "Thank God, I hear my mother's voice once more," the words of Cross's son in response to her healing (pp. 146–47).

Mix's compilation of healing testimonies was a means of religious empowerment for other women. Through public testimony, *Faith Cures* provided a public forum for other women to voice their thoughts about faith healing and other religious matters. Such works as *Faith Cures*, moreover, encouraged women to write as a religious vocation.[112] For example, Lizzie Yetley, who identifies herself as a professor of religion, writes to an unspecified editor. Alice Ball's talent as a religious poet is demonstrated in her poem "Lost the Sound of Footsteps." Other women also considered publishing their testimonies. Louise Lockwood wrote to Sarah Mix: "I have thought of publishing my case of healing for God's glory and the encouragement of others" (p. 47).

The final section of *Faith Cures* contains a somewhat extended essay, or personal narrative, on healing by Mrs. E. H. Scott of Ocean Grove, New Jersey. A type of visionary writing, her testimonial is unlike any other in the book. Although she does not mention Mix or claim to have found healing through her, her essay is interesting for what it reveals about her religious faith, her beliefs about faith healing, and how she assumes the role of a healing practitioner herself by praying for the healing of several friends and relatives, including a Mrs. B., for whom more than one prayer is offered. Scott also alludes to an unidentified figure who could be Mix:

My eye rested upon a dear lady of superior ability, and one upon whom the Divine signet had been set within the past year; she stood head and shoulders above the rest, clothed in white robes and with a halo about her; indeed, her whole being seemed a reflex of the Divine. I asked why she stood such a tower of Strength and Beauty; and without a word He pointed to the lonely pilgrim in the solitary place. I understood it, knowing the instrument used for thus advancing this young friend into God. (p. 192)

Significantly this visionary experience appears just before the last testimony in *Faith Cures*. It is a final affirmation of faith healing, of women faith healing practitioners, and most especially of the healing ministry of Sarah Mix (pp. 187–94).

Conclusion

Sarah Mix's religious experience was rooted in nineteenth-century evangelical Protestantism, specifically the independent black church tradition where she found salvation in the AME Church before moving on to the Advent Christian Church. Like other black female preachers and evangelists of the nineteenth century, for example Jarena Lee, Amanda Berry Smith, and Rebecca Cox Jackson, she crossed denominational lines. And like Amanda Berry Smith, Sarah Mix also gained attention from white Methodists and affiliated with them as a healing evangelist, speaking at Methodist Holiness camp meetings. Mix does not mention a sanctification experience. However, given that she was a regular speaker at Cullis's faith conventions, she evidently embraced Holiness teachings.

Mix is an interesting and important figure because her religious experience, as recounted in her spiritual autobiography, places her in the tradition of nineteenth-century black women preachers and evangelists who demonstrated religious leadership and authority without the benefit of ordination from a specific denomination. Unlike other black female evangelists and preachers who faced challenges and often opposition to their right to preach from male clergy in their denominations, Sarah Mix did not have to contend with challenges to her ministry from male leaders of the faith healing movement. As mentioned earlier, both Ethan O. Allen and Charles Cullis encouraged Mix as a healing evangelist and welcomed her. Probably the only challenge to Mix's public ministry was the result of the controversial nature of faith healing itself. Such opposition, moreover, was experienced by men as well.

It is not clear from the available historical evidence why Mix did not address gender, racial, and other social issues in her writings. As an independent evangelist who relied on financial donations and sales from her writings, especially *Faith Cures*, to support her (and Edward's) ministry, she may have been reluctant to mention racial issues. And although it is possible that Mix could have had experiences of racism similar to those Amanda Berry Smith recounts in her autobiography, it is also quite likely that Mix did not encounter the overt racism Smith faced.[113]

The people with whom Mix associated, including Ethan O. Allen, Charles Cullis, W. E. Boardman, A. J. Gordon, and Carrie Judd, embraced society's poor and "dispossessed" in their ministries. Gordon and Cullis, for example, were both involved in various outreach ministries to the poor and needy. Boardman had attended Lane Theological Seminary in Cincinnati, Ohio, because of its strong support of the antislavery movement, a cause he also embraced. In view of the relationship between the Holiness and faith healing movements, Vinson Synan's argument may shed additional light on Mix's experience. He writes:

The holiness camp meetings were opportunities for
Methodists of the North and South to unite on a common
platform and to begin healing the breach caused by the
Civil War and reconstruction. Perhaps Wesley's "perfect
love" could end bitter divisions in the church and also help
in reuniting the nation.[114]

Additionally, I would argue, Sarah Mix, due to the prestige
and status she enjoyed as a faith healing practitioner, probably
had a high level of self-worth that would mitigate any feelings
of racial oppression. Most importantly, as I have previously
pointed out, Sarah Mix was a woman of deep religious faith
whose primary purpose was to fulfill her calling by God to "go
work in my vineyard today" through teaching faith healing and
praying for the sick.

Faith Cures, and Answers to Prayer establishes Sarah Mix
as an important and influential figure in the divine healing movement in late-nineteenth-century America. Her gift of healing was
recognized internationally. Although her healing ministry lasted
only seven years, cut short by her death at age fifty-one, Mix became well-known in faith-healing circles and enjoyed a thriving
ministry in her hometown, a successful itinerancy, and a healing
ministry through correspondence.

Sarah Mix also established herself as a religious writer
through her journal, *Victory Through Faith*, her autobiography,
and healing testimonials. She is part of the literary and religious
tradition of black evangelical women revivalists that includes
such women as Amanda Berry Smith, Jarena Lee, Julia Foote,
Zilpha Elaw, Rebecca Cox Jackson, and Harriet Baker. Like
these and other women whose personal journeys to ministry are
recorded in spiritual narratives, Sarah Mix also endured personal tragedy. All seven of her children died at an early age. On
the other hand, unlike Jarena Lee and Julia Foote, Sarah Mix

was neither widowed nor alienated from her husband. Sarah and Edward Mix, in fact, may be unusual as an African American couple in the nineteenth century who minister together as independent evangelicals. And, equally important, Sarah Mix is part of a broader evangelical tradition that includes Phoebe Palmer, Carrie Judd Montgomery, Jennie Smith, Mrs. Michael Baxter, Hannah Whitall Smith, and many others.

Faith Cures, and Answers to Prayer attests to the religious authority of a free African American woman who was able to fashion a flourishing public ministry without being ordained. Her calling by God to "Go work in my vineyard" was all the approval and validation she needed. Accordingly, Sarah Mix believed she should document her ministry and religious leadership. Mix wanted and deserved to be recognized along with other female healing evangelists of the time. Although Mix was often referred to as "the colored lady from Wolcottville," testimonials in *Faith Cures* suggest she transcended barriers of race, class, and Victorian gender constructions of "True Womanhood."

Finally, *Faith Cures, and Answers to Prayer* is the testament of a woman of profound and deep religious faith. Through these healing testimonies we have a clearer portrait of Sarah Mix and a better understanding of her impact on the divine healing movement and of the divine healing movement itself. We can only speculate about how her ministry might have grown had she lived longer. Writing about the ministry of Sarah and Edward Mix in the early twentieth century, Carrie Judd Montgomery wrote: "These good people have long since gone to their reward, but how precious have been the streams of blessing which were started through their ministry." [115] This statement is especially true of Sarah Mix, whose faith healing ministry brought "streams of blessing" to the many sick individuals who she helped find healing through her "prayer of faith."

Epilogue

Today faith healing remains a belief and practice in various denominations, especially those that are part of the Holiness, charismatic, and Pentecostal traditions.[116] Prayer and healing, as well as the mind-body-spirit relationship, are taken seriously by believers in various religious traditions, by nonbelievers, and by physicians, scientists, and researchers.[117] One of the leading proponents of prayer and healing is Dr. Larry Dossey, the author of several books including *Healing Words: The Power of Prayer and The Practice of Medicine*.[118] Debbie Perlman, an occupational therapist and Resident Psalmist at Beth Emet The Free Synagogue, in Evanston, Illinois, maintains a website, HealingPsalm.com, where one can post names of people who are ill and need prayer. She describes her website as "a place for people of all faiths to find resources for prayer and spiritual support in times of illness." Perlman has also published a book of psalms, *Flames To Heaven: New Psalms for Healing & Praise*. "These words," she writes, "strengthen my faith in my ability to weave a lasting thread in the pattern of holiness, bound tightly to God's design."[119]

As an African American woman, I was deeply moved by and gratified to read about the Reverend Diane Lacy Winley, an African American woman who, at the time, was the coordinator of the Wellness Center at Riverside Church in New York City. "Based on God's call to wholeness," its website states, "the Wellness Center is committed to helping the congregation and community attain and maintain high level wellness and explore the many dimensions of healing for body, mind and spirit." As the website indicates, the center offers a wide range of health and wellness programs from "The Healer Within, QiGong" to a Sunday morning program of contemplative prayer, "Morning Light."[120]

In a photograph Winley is shown with another African American woman at a Sunday morning "laying on of hands" service in a chapel at Riverside Church. To move from Sarah Mix to the Reverend Winley is to move from an historical period in which the prayer of faith and laying on of hands impacted the lives of countless evangelical Americans, especially women, to a period in which that ancient rite is still meaningful. And, as most of the congregants at Winley's healing service are women, to move from Sarah Mix's era to our time is to recognize African American women's persistent religious faith and their belief in the power of prayer and the laying on of hands for healing.

Notes

1. Mrs. G. A. Wilton, "A Letter From Mrs. Wilton," in *Faith Cures, and Answers to Prayer*, by Mrs. Edward Mix (Springfield, Mass.: Press of Springfield Printing Co., 1882), 181. In quoting from *Faith Cures, and Answers to Prayer* and *The Life of Mrs. Edward Mix, Written by Herself*, I have retained the original spelling and punctuation.

2. Paul Chappell refers to her as Elizabeth. The source of the name Elizabeth is unknown. In *Faith Cures, and Answers to Prayer*, Sarah Mix is referred to as Mrs. Mix and Mrs. Edward Mix.

3. W. E. Warner defines faith healing as: "A practice, particularly associated with the Pentecostal and charismatic movements, based on the belief that Jesus' promise of healing recorded in Mark 16:18 is for every generation of believers." See W. E. Warner, "Faith Healing," in *Dictionary of Christianity in America*, ed. Daniel G. Reid (Downers Grove, Ill.: InterVarsity Press, 1990), 424. Mark 16:17–18 was one of two scriptural passages that provided a biblical basis for proponents and practitioners of faith healing in the nineteenth century: "And these signs will accompany those who believe: by using my name they will cast out demons; they will speak in new tongues; they will pick up snakes in their hands, and if they drink any deadly thing, it will not hurt them; they will lay their hands on the sick, and they will recover" (New Revised

Standard Version [NRSV]). The other passage is James 5:14–15: "Are any among you sick? They should call for the elders of the church and have them pray over them, anointing them with oil in the name of the Lord. The prayer of faith will save the sick, and the Lord will raise them up; and anyone who has committed sins will be forgiven" (NRSV).

4. See Randall K. Burkett, Nancy Hall Burkett, and Henry Louis Gates, Jr., eds. *Black Biography 1790–1950: A Cumulative Index*, vol. 2 (Alexandria, Va.: Chadwyck-Healy, Inc., 1991), 18. In this biographical entry, Edward Mix is listed as a "religious worker"; his religion is listed as Baptist.

5. *Victory Through Faith* was published monthly by the Press of Register Printing Co., Torrington, Connecticut. Mrs. Edward Mix is listed as editor and publisher. There is only one known extant issue (vol. 2, May 1884), and this is in the file on Sarah Mix at the Torrington Historical Society. The issue includes advertisements for the second edition of *In God We Trust* and *Faith Cures, and Answers to Prayer.*

6. The National Union Catalog lists the title as *In Memory of Departed Worth. The Life of Mrs. Edward Mix, Written by herself in 1880. With Appendix* (Torrington, Conn.: Press of Register Printing Co., 1884).

7. Among many useful sources on the Holiness movement are Melvin Easterday Dieter, *The Holiness Revival of the Nineteenth Century* (Metuchen, N.J.: The Scarecrow Press, 1980); Charles E. Jones, *Perfectionist Persuasion: The Holiness Movement and American Methodism, 1867–1936* (Metuchen, N.J.: The Scarecrow Press, 1974); Timothy L. Smith, "The Holiness Crusade," in *The History of American Methodism*, vol. 2, ed. Emory Stevens Bucke (New York: Abingdon Press, 1964), 608–27; Jean Miller Schmidt, "Holiness and Perfection," in *Encyclopedia of the American Religious Experience: Studies of Traditions and Movements*, vol. 2, ed. Charles H. Lippy and Peter S. Williams (New York: Charles Scribner's Sons, 1988), 813–29; Vinson Synan, *The Holiness-Pentecostal Tradition: Charismatic Movements in the Twentieth Century*, 2d. ed. (Grand Rapids, Mich.: William B. Eerdmans Publishing Co., 1997), 1–83. For sources on women and the Holiness movement see Nancy Hardesty, Lucille Sider Dayton, and Donald W. Dayton, "Women in the Holiness Movement: Feminism in the Evangeli-

cal Tradition," in *Women of Spirit: Female Leadership in the Jewish and Christian Traditions*, ed. Rosemary Radford Ruether and Eleanor T. Mclaughlin (New York: Simon and Schuster, 1979); Nancy A. Hardesty, "Evangelical Women," in *In Our Own Voices: Four Centuries of American Women's Religious Writing*, ed. Rosemary Radford Ruether and Rosemary Skinner Keller (New York: HarperSanFrancisco, 1995); Lucille Sider Dayton and Donald W. Dayton, " 'Your Daughters Shall Prophesy': Feminism in the Holiness Movement," *Methodist History* 14 (1976): 67–92. For helpful sources on black women and the Holiness movement see Adrienne M. Israel, *Amanda Berry Smith: From Washerwoman to Evangelist* (Latham, Md.: The Scarecrow Press, Inc., 1998); William L. Andrews, ed., *Sisters of the Spirit: Three Black Women's Autobiographies of the Nineteenth Century* (Bloomington: Indiana Univ. Press, 1986); Jean McMahon Humez, ed., *Gifts of Power: The Writings of Rebecca Jackson, Black Visionary, Shaker Eldress* (Amherst: Univ. of Massachusetts Press, 1981), 2–10. There has been no systematic study of blacks in the nineteenth-century Holiness movement. For information about the Holiness crusade in the black Methodist churches, see David Daniels, "Pentecostalism," in *Encyclopedia of African American Religions*, ed. Larry Murphy, J. Gordon Melton, and Gary L. Ward (New York: Garland Publishing, Inc., 1993), 585–95.

8. The result of Christian perfection, according to Wesley, was "perfect love of God and neighbor." And, moreover, one who experienced perfection was free from outward sin. Wesley's views, as has been pointed out, are often misunderstood. See "Sermon XXV, Christian Perfection," in *John Wesley's Fifty-Three Sermons*, ed. Edward H. Sugden (Nashville, Tenn.: Abingdon Press, 1983), 505–29; see also Gerald O. McCulloh, "The Call to Christian Perfection," in *The History of American Methodism*, vol. 2, ed. Emory Stevens Bucke (New York: Abingdon Press, 1964), 606–8. The Oberlin Perfectionism of revivalist Charles Grandison Finney (1792–1875) and Asa Mahan (1799–1889), Finney's associate and president of Oberlin College, was another interpretation of Wesley's doctrine of sanctification. According to this doctrine, holiness involved perfection of the will and was available to every Christian following conversion. By 1870 Mahan, the chief architect of Oberlin Perfectionism, changed his views to reflect the theology of the Higher

Christian Life Movement. See Schmidt, "Holiness and Perfection," 816–17; Edward H. Madden and James E. Hamilton, *Freedom and Grace: The Life of Asa Mahan* (Metuchen, N.J.: The Scarecrow Press, 1982).

9. For excellent studies on Phoebe Palmer's life and theology, see Charles Edward White, *The Beauty of Holiness: Phoebe Palmer as Theologian, Revivalist, Feminist, and Humanitarian* (Grand Rapids, Mich.: Francis Asbury Press of Zondervan Publishing House, 1986); Thomas C. Oden, ed., *Phoebe Palmer: Selected Writings* (New York: Paulist Press, 1988); Anne C. Loveland, "Domesticity and Religion in the Antebellum Period: The Career of Phoebe Palmer," *The Historian* 39 (May 1977): 455–71; Theodore Hovet, "Phoebe Palmer's 'Altar Phraseology' and the Spiritual Dimension of Woman's Sphere," *Journal of Religion* 63 (1983): 264–80; Margaret McFadden, "The Ironies of Pentecost: Phoebe Palmer, World Evangelism, and Female Networks," *Methodist History* 31: 63–75. Jean Miller Schmidt includes a chapter on Phoebe Palmer and Amanda Berry Smith in *Grace Sufficient: A History of Women in American Methodism, 1760–1939* (Nashville, Tenn.: Abingdon Press, 1999). Additional works on women and religion in America that give attention both to the Holiness movement and to Phoebe Palmer include Marilyn J. Westerkamp, *Women and Religion in Early America, 1600–1850: The Puritan and Evangelical Traditions* (London: Routledge, 1999), especially 104–54; Susan Hill Lindley, *"You Have Stept Out of Your Place": A History of Women and Religion in America* (Louisville, Ky.: Westminster John Knox Press, 1996); Ann Taves, *Fits, Trances, and Visions: Experiencing Religion and Explaining Experience from Wesley to James* (Princeton, N.J.: Princeton Univ. Press, 1999), 148–53.

10. In 1839 Reverend Timothy Merritt founded the *Guide to Christian Perfection*. As editor, Merritt especially requested that women contribute accounts of their experiences of sancification. Phoebe Palmer became a regular contributor to the journal. In 1845 its name was changed to *Guide to Holiness*. In 1858 Phoebe's husband, Walter Clarke Palmer, Jr., purchased it. Phoebe Palmer served as editor the last decade of her life. See Schmidt, "Holiness and Perfection," 815–16. For information on the *Guide to Holiness* see Mark Fackler and Charles H.

Lippy, eds. *Popular Religious Magazines of the United States* (West-
port, Conn.: Greenwood Press, 1995), 256–61.

11. Prayer, Bible study, and testimony characterized the Tuesday
Meeting. Begun in 1836 by Sarah A. Lankford, Phoebe Palmer's sister,
the Tuesday Meeting combined two prayer meetings Lankford led for
women of the Allen Street and Mulberry Methodist Episcopal Churches.
The Tuesday Meeting met in the home shared by Phoebe and Walter
Palmer and Sarah and Thomas Lankford. Phoebe Palmer assumed lead-
ership when the Lankfords left New York City in 1840. After Phoebe
Palmer's death in 1874, the widowed Sarah Lankford married Walter
Palmer and once again led the Tuesday Meeting until her death in 1896.

12. Phoebe, along with her husband Walter, was also influential
among British and Canadian evangelicals. The Palmers' Canadian mission began in 1853 and ended in 1859. The couple traveled to England,
Scotland, Wales, and Ireland between 1859 and 1863. In Canada, they
became prominent among British evangelicals.

13. See Schmidt, "Holiness and Perfection," 814–16.

14. Schmidt, *Grace Sufficient*, 145–47.

15. Charles Grandison Finney, the eminent nineteenth-century revivalist who later became known as "the father of modern revivalism,"
developed revival methods, or "new measures," to promote religious
conversions. He outlined this new form of revivalism in his book *Lectures on Revivals of Religion* (1835). Finney's new measures included
praying for persons in the audience by name and the protracted meeting, religious services held over several weeks and months. Finney also
pioneered the use of the "anxious bench" and "anxious meeting" for po-
tential converts. Most significantly, Finney permitted women to testify
and pray in public. See William G. McLoughlin, Jr., *Modern Revivalism:
Charles Grandison Finney to Billy Graham* (New York: Ronald Press,
1959), 85–100, and Sydney Ahlstrom, *A Religious History of the American People*, vol. 1 (Garden City, N.Y.: Image Books, 1975), 555–58. For
information about Finney and women see Nancy A. Hardesty, *"Your
Daughter Shall Prophesy": Revivalism and Feminism in the Age of
Finney* (Brooklyn, N.Y.: Carlson Publishing, 1991).

16. Schmidt, "Holiness and Perfection," 815.

17. The Christian and Missionary Alliance was founded in 1897 by

A. B. Simpson; the Church of God (Anderson, Indiana) was founded in 1881 by Daniel S. Warner; and the Salvation Army, begun in London, England, by William Booth, sent its first missionaries to the United States in 1880.

18. My historical overview of the divine healing movement relies on Paul Gale Chappell's exhaustive study, which is indispensable to an understanding of the movement. See Paul Gale Chappell, "The Divine Healing Movement in America" (Ph.D. diss., Drew Univ., 1983). Chappell describes adherents of the divine healing movement as "that group of persons who maintain the belief that physical disease or illness is cured by the supernatural intervention of God when the prayer of faith is prayed," v, 81–86. See also Donald W. Dayton, *Theological Roots of Pentecostalism* (Grand Rapids, Mich.: Francis Asbury Press, 1987), chap. 5; and Raymond J. Cunningham, "From Holiness to Healing: The Faith Cure in America 1872–1892," *Church History* 43 (1972): 499–513. In my introduction I use faith cure, faith healing, and divine healing interchangeably as their nineteenth-century adherents and practitioners did. Also, I do not include material on John Alexander Dowie and faith healing in Pentecostalism, both of which are more important to the history of faith healing in the twentieth century. This material is included in Chappell and in David Edwin Harrell, Jr., *All Things Are Possible: The Healing and Charismatic Revivals in Modern America* (Bloomington: Indiana Univ. Press, 1975).

19. See Chappell, "The Divine Healing Movement," 88–89, 89–91 n. 4. Along with recording various healings in his journal, Wesley wrote two books espousing his teaching on health and his theological views on pain and sickness. For discussions of health, healing, and medicine in Methodism, see Harold Y. Vanderpool, "The Wesleyan-Methodist Tradition," in *Caring and Curing: Health and Medicine in the Western Religious Traditions*, ed. Ronald L. Numbers and Darrel W. Amundsen (New York: Macmillan Publishing Co., 1986), 317–53; E. Brooks Holifield, *Health and Medicine in the Methodist Tradition: Journey Toward Wholeness* (New York: The Crossroad Publishing Co., 1986).

20. For a biographical sketch of Ethan Otis Allen, see Chappell, "The Divine Healing Movement," 87–104. Chappell has provided abundant biographical information and extensively documented the min-

istries of the primary leaders in the divine healing movement through an examination of their writings and contemporary popular religious literature.

21. Ibid., 92 n. 7.

22. The ministry of Sarah and Edward Mix is discussed in Chappell, "The Divine Healing Movement," 92–98. I am grateful to Nancy Hardesty for allowing me to read her unpublished essay on Sarah Mix, "Holiness and Healing: A Nineteenth-Century Case Study" and for information on Mix's family background from the *Winsted and Torrington Directory*. This information is available in a file on Sarah Mix at the Torrington Historical Society, Torrington, Connecticut.

23. Faith healing, specifically the practice of praying for the sick and laying on of hands, had occurred as early as 1672 when George Fox, founder of the Society of Friends, conducted a missionary tour in colonial America. Other religious groups, including the Shakers, the Mormons, the Oneida Community, and Seventh-day Adventists under the leadership of health reformer Ellen G. Harmon White, also practiced faith healing. Chappell discusses early influences from the seventeenth through the early nineteenth centuries along with European influences in his study. See Chappell, "The Divine Healing Movement," 1–57. Simpson, Gordon, and Boardman are also known by their full names: Albert Benjamin Simpson, Adoniram Judson Gordon, and William E. Boardman.

24. All aspects of Cullis's ministry are discussed in Chappell, "The Divine Healing Movement," 104–91. Following his death in 1892, Cullis's various faith works suffered and ended in 1899. Cullis's faith healing homes, however, closed shortly after his death as few individuals came. Ibid., 189–91.

25. Lucy Drake's dramatic healing catapulted her into public ministry in the Holiness and faith healing movements. After her healing, she conducted Cullis's first foreign missionary venture. Her healing so inspired W. E. Boardman, who was yet to promote faith healing publicly, that he invited her to speak at his holiness conventions, where she testified of her healing through the ministry of Cullis. Drake (later known as Lucy Drake Osborne) also operated a faith cure home. Chappell, "The Divine Healing Movement," 129, 199.

26. These were Methodist-owned camp meeting sites used for Holiness camp meetings. In order to have more flexibility in planning his conventions, Cullis purchased his own property.

27. Chappell, "The Divine Healing Movement," 152–56. Cullis also held winter conventions in Boston and held faith conventions in such major cities as Chicago, Baltimore, Philadelphia, and New York.

28. Ibid., 84–85; 85 n. 165.

29. Cullis published two additional volumes: *More Faith Cures; or Answers to Prayer in the Healing of the Sick* (1881) and *Other Faith Cures; or Answers to Prayer in the Healing of the Sick* (1885). Both volumes were published by the Willard Tract Repository. These books, the first of their kind, included healing testimonies. As Chappell notes: "Cullis' purpose in publishing these testimonies was to show Christians that God still honored his promises, that He was still in living commerce with his creation" (139). Cullis also published an *Annual Report*, which basically gave a financial accounting of the ministry and was the means by which Cullis obtained funds to support his faith work. Before these publications on faith healing, Cullis founded and published a magazine on Holiness, *Times of Refreshing* (1869), as well as two other monthly magazines: *The Word of Life* (1874), targeted to unbelievers, and, for children, *Loving Words* (1874); Chappell, "The Divine Healing Movement," 119–22.

30. See Cunningham, "From Holiness to Healing," 503. Cullis's publishing house, like his faith conventions, became so successful that it expanded to include branches in New York City, London, California, and other places. Chappell, "The Divine Healing Movement," 121–22.

31. Ibid., 105.

32. W. E. Boardman, *The Higher Christian Life* (Boston: Henry Hoyt, 1859); *Faith Work Under Dr. Cullis, in Boston* (Boston: Willard Tract Repository, 1874).

33. Boardman returned briefly to the United States before making England his permanent home in December 1875. The Higher Christian Life movement originated in America among evangelical Protestants active in the Holiness movement in the late nineteenth century. It became internatinal through the Keswick Movement. Named for a village in northwest England, the Keswick Movement held annual conventions

devoted to fostering the "higher Christian life," or the "victorious life," beginning in 1875. Although a product of the American Holiness movement, the Keswick Movement developed its own unique theology and emphases. Based in the theology of the Reformed tradition, the Keswick movement stressed gradual, as opposed to immediate, sanctification. Keswick theology also emphasized the "suppression" rather than the eradication of sin. William and Mary Boardman and Robert and Hannah Whitall Smith were essential to the development of the Keswick movement. They were popular speakers at Keswick conventions and their books were well-known in England. In addition to Boardman's *The Higher Christian Life* (1859), Robert Pearsall Smith's *Holiness Through Faith* (1870) and Hannah Whitall Smith's *The Christian's Secret of a Happy Life* (1875), published by Cullis, disseminated Keswick Holiness teaching. In the 1880s revivalist Dwight L. Moody (1837–1899) brought Keswick Holiness back to the United States in his Northfield conferences. See Steven Barabas, *So Great Salvation: The History and Messages of the Keswick Convention* (Westwood, N.J.: Fleming H. Revell, 1952); George M. Marsden, *Fundamentalism and American Culture: The Shaping of Twentieth-Century Evangelicism: 1870–1925* (New York: Oxford Univ. Press, 1980); Schmidt, "Holiness and Perfection," 820–21.

34.　Chappell, "The Divine Healing Movement," 193–204; *The Great Physician (Jehovah Rophi)* (Boston: Willard Tract Repository, 1881). Although Chappell cites this work as *The Lord That Healeth Thee (Jehovah Rophi)*, the title for the English edition, published in London in 1881, I use *The Great Physician* in referring to this work.

35.　Three female supporters, Charlotte Murray, Elizabeth Sisson, and Mrs. Michael Baxter, bought and furnished the home and served as its matrons. Baxter and Murray were prolific writers whose works helped spread the doctrine of faith healing both in Europe and in America. Baxter and her husband, the founder and editor of the *Christian Herald* (London) and the *Christian Magazine* (New York), publicized Boardman's healing ministry and Bethshan in their periodicals. Sisson had found healing through Charles Cullis's ministry and received training in his deaconess home. In the 1890s Sisson returned to America and united with Carrie Judd's healing ministry. She became associate editor of *Triumphs of Faith*, the periodical Judd founded and edited. Chappell, "The Divine Healing Movement," 203–9.

36. Chappell, "The Divine Healing Movement," 250–77.

37. Ibid., 266 n. 187.

38. A. B. Simpson, *The Gospel of Healing* (New York: Christian Alliance Publishing, 1896); Chappell, "The Divine Healing Movement," 272–76.

39. A. J. Gordon, *The Ministry of Healing: Miracles of Cure in All Ages*, 2d ed. (Harrisburg, Pa.: Christian Publications, 1961); Chappell, "The Divine Healing Movement," 219–28, 226 n. 88.

40. Ibid., 159–60.

41. J. M. Buckley, *Faith-Healing, Christian Science and Kindred Phenomena* (New York: The Century Co., 1898), 45–46.

42. R. (Captain Robert) Kelso Carter, who found healing for a heart condition through Cullis's prayers, was a friend and enthusiastic supporter of Cullis. He wrote one of the first theological statements on faith healing in a book published by Cullis's Willard Tract Repository, *The Atonement for Sin and Sickness; or a Full Salvation for Body and Soul* (1884). Carter reformulated his theological views in *"Faith Healing" Reviewed After Twenty Years* (Boston: The Christian Witness Co., 1897).

43. Chappell, "The Divine Healing Movement," 202.

44. Ibid., 170–71.

45. Ibid., 226 n. 88.

46. Ibid., 228.

47. Ibid., 224.

48. Ibid., 141, 280. Cullis, who provided free medical services and prescriptions to the poor, did not object to the use of medicine. Simpson and Boardman, on the other hand, objected to the use of medicine.

49. Chappell, "The Divine Healing Movement," 104, 176; Ethan O. Allen, *Faith Healing: or, What I Have Witnessed of the Fulfillment of James V: 14, 15, 16* (Philadelphia, 1881).

50. Ibid., 166–69. Opposition accompanied the increase in faith homes.

51. Carrie Judd, "Faith-Rest Cottage," *Triumphs of Faith* 2 (May 1882): 71. This aspect of Judd's ministry began first as a "Faith Sanctu-

ary," the parlor in her family home devoted to weekly "faith-meetings," in which prayer for the sick was offered. In 1881 she began renting a two-story frame cottage in her neighborhood and purchased the property one year later. See Carrie Judd, "Faith-Rest Cottage," *Triumphs of Faith* (Feb. 1882): 19–20; "Faith-Rest Cottage," *Triumphs of Faith* (Apr. 1882): 59–60.

52. Carrie Judd, "Faith-Rest Cottage," *Triumphs of Faith* 2 (July 1882): 107.

53. Chappell, "The Divine Healing Movement," 166–67. Chappell includes the names of ten homes operated by women during the early 1880s, including Lucy Drake Osborn's Home for Incurables in Brooklyn, N.Y., and Carrie Judd's Faith-Rest Cottage in Buffalo, N.Y. The most popular faith homes were Judd's Faith-Rest Cottage (1882), Charles Cullis's faith home (1882), and A. B. Simson's Berachah Home (1884).

54. Ibid., 183. The complete title of Judd's journal was *Triumphs of Faith: A Monthly Journal, Devoted to Faith-Healing, and to the Promotion of Christian Holiness*. It was published until 1979. Judd's *The Prayer of Faith* and *"Under His Wings"* (1936) have been reprinted and published in Donald W. Dayton, ed., *The Life and Teachings of Carrie Judd Montgomery* (New York: Garland Publishing, Inc., 1985).

55. Chappell, "The Divine Healing Movement," 183 n. 223.

56. Ibid., 205–6.

57. Ibid., 234–35.

58. Ibid., 99.

59. Ibid., 229–50. In 1890 Carrie Judd married George S. Montgomery. She closed Faith-Rest Cottage when they moved to Oakland, California. In 1893 the Montgomerys opened a new faith home, the Home of Peace, which continued operating even after Judd's death in 1946.

60. Ibid., 175, 183–86.

61. Buckley, *Faith-Healing, Christian Science and Kindred Phenomena*, 6. For another perspective on Buckley, see Taves, *Fits, Trances, and Visions* , especially 226–32.

62. Chappell, "The Divine Healing Movement," 363.

63. Cunningham, "From Holiness to Healing," 512–13.

64. Gail Parker offers a useful definition of mind cure, which she

uses "in a generic sense to refer to a faith (and the practices growing out of it) in the power of mind over body, and, more specifically, in the power to heal oneself through right thinking." See Gail Parker, *Mind Cure in New England: From the Civil War to World War I* (Hanover, N.H.: Univ. Press of New England, 1973), ix.

65. J. Gordon Melton, "Christian Science-Metaphysical Family," in *Encyclopedia of American Religions*, 3 vols. (Tarrytown, N.Y.: Triumph Books, 1991), 2:133–39.

66. Robert Peel, *Mary Baker Eddy: The Years of Discovery* (New York: Holt, Rinehart and Winston, 1966), 197.

67. Ibid., 197.

68. Prologue to "Christian Science in Tremont Temple," in *The Emergence of Christian Science In American Religious Life*, by Stephen Gottschalk (Berkeley: Univ. of California Press, 1973), xv-xxix, especially xxi. Tremont Temple was an important center of revivalism and Holiness evangelism in Boston. Chappell, "The Divine Healing Movement," 114 n. 57.

69. Mary Baker Eddy, *Miscellaneous Writings, 1883–1896* (Boston: Trustees under the Will of Mary Baker G. Eddy, 1896), 96.

70. Gottschalk, *The Emergence of Christian Science*, 226.

71. Mary Baker Eddy, *Science and Health with Key to the Scriptures* (Boston: Trustees under the Will of Mary Baker G. Eddy, 1910), 1, quoted in Gottschalk, *The Emergence of Christian Science*, 226.

72. Eddy, *Miscellaneous Writings*, 43.

73. Mary Baker Eddy, *Manual of The Mother Church* (Boston: Trustees under the Will of Mary Baker G. Eddy, 1919), 47, quoted in Gottschalk, *The Emergence of Christian Science*, 221.

74. Chappell, "The Divine Healing Movement," 359.

75. Ibid., 361.

76. Taves, *Fits, Trances, and Visions*, 4.

77. Frank S. Townsend, "Faith-Cure," *Christian Advocate* 57 (1882): 660, quoted in Chappell, "The Divine Healing Movement," 153.

78. Albert J. Raboteau, "The Afro-American Traditions," in *Caring and Curing: Health and Medicine in the Western Religious Traditions*, ed. Ronald L. Numbers and Darrel W. Amundsen (New York: Macmillan Publishing Co., 1986), 539–62; Albert J. Raboteau, *Slave Reli-*

gion: The "Invisible Institution" in the Antebellum South (New York: Oxford Univ. Press, 1978), 275–88. For a related discussion, see Yvonne Chireau, "Conjure and Christianity in the Nineteenth Century: Religious Elements in African American Magic," *Religion and American Culture: A Journal of Interpretation* 7 (Summer 1997): 225–46.

79. See Raboteau, "The Afro-American Traditions," 554–56.

80. Albert J. Raboteau, introduction to *God Struck Me Dead: Voices of Ex-Slaves*, ed. Clifton H. Johnson (Cleveland, Ohio: The Pilgrim Press, 1993), 60, quoted in Sharla Fett, " 'It's a Spirit in Me': Spiritual Power and the Healing Work of African American Women in Slavery," in *A Mighty Baptism: Race, Gender, and the Creation of American Protestantism*, ed. Susan Juster and Lisa MacFarlane (Ithaca: Cornell Univ. Press, 1996), 189–190. Other useful studies on slave women and healing include Martia Graham Goodson, "Medical-Botanical Contributions of African Slave Women to American Medicine," *The Western Journal of Black Studies* 11: 198–203; Yvonne Chireau, "The Uses of the Supernatural: Toward a History of Black Women's Magical Practices," in Juster and MacFarlane, *A Mighty Baptism*, 171–88.

81. Henry Louis Gates, Jr., ed. *An Autobiography: The Story of the Lord's Dealings with Mrs. Amanda Smith the Colored Evangelist* (New York: Oxford Univ. Press, 1988), 99.

82. Fett, " 'It's a Spirit in Me,' " 189–209.

83. Ibid., 198.

84. See Jon Butler, *Awash in a Sea of Faith: Christianizing the American People* (Cambridge, Mass.: Harvard Univ. Press, 1990), 67–97, 151–53; Mechal Sobel, *The World They Made Together: Black and White Values in Eighteenth-Century Virginia* (Princeton, N.J.: Princeton Univ. Press, 1987).

85. Fett, " 'It's a Spirit in Me,' " 192.

86. Raboteau, "The Afro-American Traditions," 544.

87. Sarah Mix's spiritual autobiography follows the pattern of American spiritual autobiography written by evangelical women and men, black and white. These narratives emphasized the soul's journey from damnation to salvation. In her study of women's conversion narratives Virginia Brereton enumerates five stages of the conversion

process that are found in the "classic" nineteenth-century narrative: life before the onset of the conversion process; an awareness of one's sinfulness and the possibility of eternal damnation; yielding to God in conversion; changes in behavior and attitudes as a result of conversion; and descriptions of times of discouragement followed by rededication. See Virginia Lieson Brereton, *From Sin to Salvation: Stories of Women's Conversions, 1800 to the Present* (Bloomington: Indiana Univ. Press, 1991), 6.

88. Andrews, *Sisters of the Spirit*, 11.

89. It appears that the Mixes remained members of the Advent Christian Church in Torrington. Organized in 1860, the Advent Christian Church grew out of the Millerite movement of the 1830s and 1840s. Sarah Mix's obituary in *Victory Through Faith* was written by the Reverend Frank H. Burbank, who also delivered the eulogy at her funeral. Nancy Hardesty indicates that Burbank may have been the supply pastor for the Advent Christian Church.

90. See Humez, *Gifts of Power*. See also Nellie Y. McKay, "Nineteenth-Century Black Women's Spiritual Autobiographies: Religious Faith and Self-Empowerment," in *Interpreting Women's Lives: Feminist Theory and Personal Narratives* ed. Personal Narratives Group (Bloomington: Indiana Univ. Press, 1989), 139–54.

91. Andrews, *Sisters of the Spirit*, 11.

92. Although Allen used "gift of healing" to refer to Mix's religious vocation, Mix viewed herself as a woman of prayer and faith, not as a healer per se. Mix and other healing evangelists of this period did not refer to themselves as healers. Rather they viewed themselves mainly as people of prayer who prayed with the sick and sometimes, in faithfulness to the biblical command in James 5:14, anointed with oil and laid hands on the sick person. This self-understanding differs markedly from that of Maria B. Woodworth-Etter, Aimee Semple McPherson, and other early-twentieth-century preachers and evangelists who viewed themselves as healers who have healing power and a gift of healing that others do not have. I am grateful to Nancy Hardesty for calling the distinction to my attention.

93. See Chappell, "The Divine Healing Movement," 92–97. The

Mixes encountered opposition to their faith healing ministry. Sarah Mix tried to get support for their ministry, and faith healing in general, through her writings on faith healing. Her views were published in *Triumphs of Faith* and in her own journal and in *Faith Cures*. Although Chappell devotes six consecutive pages to the ministry of Sarah and Edward Mix and mentions Sarah Mix in a section on women's participation in the divine healing movement, he does not cite her writings. He relies primarily, it seems, for information about Mix from Judd's publications as well as Buckley's article on Mix.

94. See Randall K. Burkett, Nancy Hall Burkett, and Henry Louis Gates, Jr., eds., "Pastor Henry N. Jeter's Twenty-five Years Experience with the Shiloh Baptist Church and Her History," in *Black Biographical Dictionaries 1790–1950* (Alexandria, Va.: Chadwyck-Healy, Inc., 1987), microfiche.

95. Edward M. Mix, "To Our Readers," *Victory Through Faith* 2 (May 1884): 38.

96. The entire text is reprinted in Andrews, *Sisters of the Spirit*, 25–48. For additional discussion of Lee's text, see also Frances Smith Foster, *Written by Herself: Literary Production by African American Women, 1746–1892* (Bloomington: Indiana Univ. Press, 1993), 56–75.

97. Chappell, "The Divine Healing Movement," 92–93.

98. See Foster, *Written by Herself*, 181.

99. Sarah Mix theologized, like other evangelical women, black and white, in the nineteenth century. It is appropriate to call her a "lay theologian," because she apparently had no formal academic training in theology. In her study of black Baptist women, particularly Virginia Broughton, Mary Cook, and Lucy Wilmot Smith, Evelyn Brooks Higginbotham points out that the act of theologizing was not limited to male clergy or to college-educated women. Many women belonged to Bible Bands and recited and interpreted scriptural passages at their meetings. See Evelyn Brooks Higginbotham, *Righteous Discontent: The Women's Movement in the Black Baptist Church 1880–1920* (Cambridge, Mass.: Harvard Univ. Press, 1993), 120–49. For a related discussion, see Humez, *Gifts of Power*, 4–7.

100. According to Gail Kruppa, archivist at the Torrington Historical

Society, Wolcottville was the center of the town Torrington. At the turn of the century, Wolcottville was no longer used as a geographical designation. (Phone query Oct. 19, 2000).

101. Not using medicine was a controversial practice, not only with Mix, but with other faith healers as well, and the source of much opposition and hostility.

102. In her unpublished essay "Holiness and the Rhetoric of Healing: Two Case Studies," Nancy Hardesty provides information on Jennie Smith, who claimed spiritual healing from a physical condition that left her unable to walk. Smith published several books about her life and traveled as an evangelist. "She called herself the 'Railroad Evangelist' because, since her cot required her to travel in the baggage car, she often had opportunity to bear Christian witness to trainmen who assisted her." I am grateful to Nancy Hardesty for sharing this essay with me.

103. See Daniel E. Albrecht, "Carrie Judd Montgomery: Pioneering Contributor to Three Religious Movements," *Pneuma: The Journal of the Society for Pentecostal Studies* (1986): 101–19. Carrie Judd's ministry spanned the Holiness, divine healing, and Pentecostal movements. Although she began her ministry as a Holiness lay person through her association with the Christian and Missionary Alliance, she joined the Assemblies of God in 1917. Interestingly, Albrecht refers to Mix as an "obscure healer."

104. During her extended recovery, Judd also asked Charles Cullis to pray for her complete restoration to health. Interestingly, in her testimony in Mix's book, a paragraph is omitted that appears in her testimony in the prayer of faith: "I wish to add that Dr. Charles Cullis, of Boston, Mass., whose faith-works and faith cures are so widely known, kindly added his prayers for my complete recovery." See Judd, *The Prayer of Faith*, 19.

105. Maria B. Woodworth-Etter was affiliated with the United Brethren from 1880 to 1884 and the Churches of God from 1884 to 1904. She then announced that she was an independent evangelist, although she generally associated with Pentecostal congregations. In 1885 in a revival in Hartford City, Ind., Woodworth-Etter began the practice of praying for the sick and within a short time demonstrated her effectiveness as a healing evangelist. In 1890 Carrie Judd Montgomery met

Woodworth-Etter in Oakland, Calif., where they were both conducting healing revivals, and the two remained friends and colleagues until Woodworth-Etter's death. Her faith healing ministry, however, led to legal problems in 1913, 1915, and 1920. She faced charges of practicing medicine without a license and eliciting funds under false pretenses. Despite her legal problems and controversy surrounding her ministry, Woodworth-Etter was a shining example for Aimee Semple McPherson, whose persistent hope of meeting her was finally fulfilled in Indianapolis in 1918. For a general introduction to the life of Maria Woodworth-Etter, see Wayne E. Warner, *The Woman Evangelist: The Life and Times of Charismatic Evangelist Maria B. Woodworth-Etter* (Metuchen, N.J.: The Scarecrow Press, 1986). See also Edith L Blumhofer, *Aimee Semple McPherson: Everybody's Sister* (Grand Rapids, Mich.: William B. Eerdmans, 1993), 140.

106. Chappell, "The Divine Healing Movement," 249.

107. Judd, *"Under His Wings,"* 60.

108. Andrews, *Sisters of the Spirit*, 3. In describing the relationship between Jarena Lee and Zilpha Elaw, William Andrews writes: "Jarena Lee welcomed Elaw into evangelism as her spiritual sister, happily sharing at least one pulpit with her. Eventually the two women's life stories would prove them literary compatriots as well."

109. Mrs. Edward Mix, "Holding Fast," *Triumphs of Faith* (1881): 4–5; Mrs. Edward Mix, "Faith in God," *Triumphs of Faith* (1881): 83. Chappell attributes "Faith Healing," published in the same journal in 1881, to Edward Mix. The author's initials E. P. M. verify that this was not written by Edward Mix, whose middle initial was M.

110. Common complaints by those seeking healing through prayer included paralysis, spinal injuries, eye problems, migraine headaches, intestinal and stomach problems, and "nervous prostration." Also, many individuals indicated in their testimonies that they had been sick for a long time and that neither the care of a physician nor medicine had effected a cure and return to health.

111. See Charles Rosenberg, "The American Medical Profession: Mid-Nineteenth Century," *Mid-America* 44 (1962): 169–70. According to Rosenberg, "Homeopathy, the most wide-spread of the medical sects competing with the medical profession, benefitted not only from this

climate of opinion, but from a rapidly increasing German immigration which provided both patients and practitioners. Like hydropathy, moreover, homeopathy was relatively inexpensive and at worst harmless." See also Martin Kaufman, "Homeopathy in America: The Rise and Fall and Persistence of a Medical Heresy," in *Other Healers: Unorthodox Medicine in America*, ed. Norman Gevitz (Baltimore, Md.: Johns Hopkins Univ. Press, 1988), 99–123.

112. Schmidt, *Grace Sufficient*, 140–41. Jean Miller Schmidt discusses writing as a religious vocation among Methodist women, especially Phoebe Palmer and Mary James, who exchanged letters as a means of offering spiritual encouragement and support to one another. Mary James, like Phoebe Palmer, also wrote poetry, hymns, and an autobiography for young people.

113. See Gates, *An Autobiography*, 94, 119. In her autobiography, Smith writes about the racism at Phoebe Palmer's Tuesday Meeting and at Kennebunk Camp Meeting. See also Nancy A. Hardesty and Adrienne Israel, "Amanda Berry Smith: A 'Downright, Outright Christian,'" in *Spiritual and Social Responsibility: Vocational Vision of Women in the United Methodist Tradition*, ed. Rosemary Skinner Keller (Nashville, Tenn.: Abingdon Press, 1993), 68–71.

114. See Synan, *The Holiness-Pentecostal Tradition*, 31.

115. Judd, *"Under His Wings,"* 60.

116. See David Edwin Harrell, Jr., *All Things Are Possible: The Healing and Charismatic Revivals in Modern America* (Bloomington: Indiana Univ. Press, 1975).

117. A good overview of these developments is Winifred Gallagher, "Seeking Help for the Body in the Well-Being of the Soul," *New York Times*, Sunday, 13 June 1999, sec. WH, p. 23.

118. Larry Dossey, *Healing Words: The Power of Prayer and The Practice of Medicine* (New York: HarperSanFrancisco, 1993).

119. Debbie Perlman, *Flames To Heaven: New Psalms for Healing & Praise* (Wilmette, Ill.: RadPublishers, 1998); see, "A Psalmist for Our Times," <www.healingpsalm.com>.

120. See Gallagher, "Seeking Help for the Body in the Well-Being of the Soul"; <www.theriversidechurch.org/programs_health.html>.

FAITH CURES,

AND

ANSWERS TO PRAYER

Mrs. EDWARD MIX

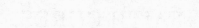

THE OLD VERSION.

"Now faith is the substance of things hoped for, the evidence of things not seen."—Heb. xi. 1.

THE NEW VERSION.

"Now faith is the assurance of things hoped for, the proving of things not seen."

"O Lord, my God, I cried unto Thee and thou hast healed me."—Psalms xxx. 2.

"And the Lord will take away from thee all sickness."—Deut. vii. 15.

"And behold there was a certain man before Him which had the dropsy, and He took him and healed him and let him go."—Luke xiv. 2–4.

"Bless the Lord, O my soul, and forget not all his benefits, who forgiveth all thine iniquities, who healeth all thy diseases."—Psalms ciii. 2, 3.

"And behold there came a Leper and worshipped Him, saying, Lord if Thou wilt Thou canst make me clean, and Jesus put forth his hand and touched him, saying, I will, be thou clean, and immediately his leprosy was cleansed."—Mat. viii. 2, 3.

"And behold there was a man which had his hand withered, then said He to the man, stretch forth thine hand, and he stretched it forth, and it was restored whole like unto the other."—Mat. xii. 10–13.

"I will put none of these diseases upon thee, for I am the Lord that healeth thee."—Exodus xv. 26.

"I have heard thy prayer, I have seen thy tears, behold I will heal thee."—2 Kings xx. 5.

PREFACE.

Does God answer prayer? Every true-hearted Christian would answer yes. What should be the nature and character of prayer? It should be offered in faith, and with a wise reference to the glory of God, and it is very necessary that the heart should be all right in the sight of God, then we can come boldly to the throne of grace and obtain mercy and grace to help in every time of need, and we can come with a full assurance of faith, for we read in God's Word, "Therefore, I say unto you what things soever ye desire, when ye pray, believe that ye receive them, and ye shall have them," and we read, "The eyes of the Lord are over the righteous, and his ears are open unto their prayers." But many who believe it is right to come to God with spiritual sickness question whether it is right to come in like manner with physical disease. All that have arrived at the age of maturity, and acknowledge God's Word to be true, believe that when Christ was here on the earth and went about doing good, he healed all manner of diseases, and raised the dead, and the same Jesus says, "All power is given to me in Heaven and in earth." But many will ask the question, how is it done? Such was the inquiry in the time of the Apostles. Turn to the third chapter of Acts, and read to the 17th verse, when the people looked with wonder and astonishment upon the one which had been a cripple from his birth, and Peter said unto him, "Silver and gold have I none, but such as I have give I thee, in the name of Jesus Christ of Nazareth rise up and walk, and immediately his ankle bones received strength." Did the man say, don't say anything about this to any one, Peter, for fear it won't last, then people would ridicule me? No; that was not his feeling at all, but he went right into the temple with them, walking and leaping, and praising God, and when the people marveled at this, Peter says, "It's through no power or holiness in us that has made this man whole," but he says, "The God of Abraham, and of Isaac, and of Jacob, the God of our fathers, hath glorified his Son Jesus, whom ye delivered up and denied him in the presence of Pilate when he was determined to let him go; his name through faith in

His name hath made this man strong, whom ye see and know, the faith which is by him hath given him this perfect soundness in the presence of you all." And I thank God to-day that the same faith, put in lively exercise, will produce the same effect.

Turn to the 11th chapter of Hebrews and see what was accomplished by faith. Is the ear of God heavier to-day, that he does not hear, or his arm shortened that he does not save? Nay, verily, he is the same yesterday, to-day, and for-ever. But, says one, we have no such spirit-ual gifts in the churches now as they used to have. Turn to the 12th chapter of 1st Corinthians and read the gifts of the church. The word says, "Now concerning spiritual gifts, brethren, I would not have you ignorant," then goes on describing the different gifts, and there is no place between the lids of the Bible where we read those gifts have ever been withdrawn; but the churches have degenerated from the truth and its proper standing so much so, that even professing Christians will call it the work of the Devil. But we that believe that the prayer of faith shall save the sick, " and the Lord shall raise him up, and if he has committed sins they shall be forgiven him," let us take courage, for they said of Christ, he hath a devil; but some said, " can a devil open the eyes of the blind?" Now God has promised, and that is enough for us; faith begins only when reasoning ends, and if we wish God to answer, stop asking questions whether He will or will not, and how. God's promises are unqualified, save that they require an unhesitating faith which asks no questions, only believes, and believing as I do, that God's promises are sure, and that by a blessed and happy experience have proved them as such, I feel it my duty to lay my experience before the public, although I consider my weakness and insufficiency to do the work, but ask God to lead my mind and guide my pen as I write, that I might increase the faith of some poor suffering ones, who are beyond the reach of aid from the arm of flesh, and are willing to trust in God for deliverance.

I was born of a consumptive family, and nearly twenty-three years ago a skillful physician after sounding my lungs, told me I could not live over two weeks; I could not go up a pair of stairs without sitting down on them once or twice; my cough was terrible, he gave me some

tincture of barks, and told me to diet and to leave
the city, and if I had any friends in the country
to go there. So I came to my sisters, in Goshen,
Conn., and following his advice I began to improve, by the change of air and rest from hard labor;
the improvement was rapid, in a few months I was
able to go out to service, and the next spring following I was married. My general health was
very good for years, I was able to do almost any
amount of labor. In the meantime loved ones were
added to the family, but only to sicken and die;
and so we have laid them away one by one, those
we loved in other years, till alone and broken-
hearted we have nothing left but tears; the last
lovely one we laid in her resting place eight
years ago, which made seven in number; all died
with lung disease. Then my health began to fail,
my lungs became very weak, and with all the
tenderness and weakness there was about them,
yet I could sing. I was growing so weak in
body that I could not walk down to the hall to
meeting. I did so dread the thought that I could
not walk that distance, which was not one quarter
of a mile, and the two last times I walked down
Mr. Mix was obliged to go home and harness the

horse and come after me. Consumption had again made its second attack. About that time sister Whitney, of Wolcottville, was very sick; she had four or five different physicians, still she was failing, there was no hope unless God interposed; I talked with brother Whitney, and finally prevailed upon him to send for brother Allen of Springfield, Mass., who I had heard had the gift of healing.

He was sent for and he came, bringing with him brother and sister Loomis; after I heard they had come I began to think about myself, and reason like this: you have so much faith that sister Whitney will be healed in answer to prayer, why don't you have brother Allen pray for you? I settled the question in my mind in this way, I would say nothing to brother Allen about it, but if he said anything about praying for me, all right.

The next morning, December 19th, 1877, after their arrival they came over to our house to have a season of prayer for sister Whitney. Mr. Mix and myself united our prayers with them in behalf of sister Whitney, and when I was praying brother Allen noticed something in my prayer that convinced him that all was not right with me concerning health, and he asked me if I enjoyed good health. I replied, no, sir; he asked me if I did not believe that God would heal me in answer to prayer, the reply was, yes; he said, do you believe he will heal you now? yes, was the quick answer; he said, all unite in prayer with me in behalf of sister Mix.

We again knelt in prayer, and as brother Allen felt the power of the Holy Ghost upon him, he arose and laid his hand upon my head, in the name of the Lord; at that moment I believed I was healed, the room was filled with the glory of God, so much so that sister Loomis fell to the floor as one dead, and I was so overwhelmed with the power of God, I felt that everything like disease was removed; I felt as light as a feather, as if I could run through a troop, and leap over a wall. I leaped for joy into the other room, shouting victory in the name of Jesus, and I was not afraid to tell it that I was healed of some troubles I had for twenty years, I was relieved of them, praise the name of the Lord. Brother Allen said he was impressed that I had the gift of healing; I could hardly believe it to be true, still it was in my mind a great deal, and as I believe in proving all things, and holding fast to that which is good, I had a

little wart under my right eye the size of a small
darning needle, I thought I would take that as a
test, and as I retired at night I told the Lord in
these words: I will lay my hand upon this in the
name of Jesus, and if I have the gift let this be
removed. As I arose in the morning, being very
busy about my household cares I did not think of
it until I was passing the mirror, I stopped, and
to my surprise it was withered and dry; I just
touched it and it dropped off. I knew it was of the
Lord. In a few days I was taken with diphtheria,
and I took it to the Lord in prayer, laying my
hand upon my throat in the name of Jesus, and in
less than a day I was entirely cured of it, and so
the Lord has led me on. I commenced laboring
among neighbors. Then the news spread to
towns and villages, and cities and states, and I can
say, praise the Lord for his goodness and his
wonderful works to the children of men.

ANSWERS TO PRAYER.

VICTORY THROUGH CHRIST.

In this chapter is given the experience of a dear sister, who has been brought triumphantly through the conflict, by the conquering might of her Lord; and before my dear readers listen to the recital of her long illness and wonderful deliverance, I believe that they will be interested in a sweet little poem, which she composed when she had no thought of being freed from her suffering, except by death. To all those who are still helpless these little verses will be a song attuned to their own heart-longings.

LOST, THE SOUND OF FOOTSTEPS.

BY ALICE M. BALL.

Lost, the sound of footsteps—my own footsteps; just once more
Do I long to hear the music of my feet upon the floor;
Dream I of the days, now vanished, when my lips first learned to talk,
Of the mother's love that fondly taught a little child to walk:
In the silence that surrounds me, tired of silence, tired of pain,
Do I long for hands to guide me till I've learned to walk again.

Lost, the sound of footsteps; how the days have come and
    gone,
And my steps, forever silenced, wake no echo in our home.
Music floats about me, sweetly wafted on the air,
And the hum of merry voices sounds about me everywhere,
While I fondly long for music, that can be mine nevermore—
Just the music of my footsteps—my own footsteps on the floor.

Lost, the sound of footsteps; and I wait, day after day,
In the midst of this long silence, where the Master bids me stay,
And dream of spacious meadows, where my child feet used to
    roam;
Of the foot-prints left so often on the graveled walks at home.
Does the Father know how restless our weak human feet may
    grow,
And does He guide them just as safely, when they lie in
    shadows so?

Lost, the sound of footsteps; when the soul's work here is done,
When the gates of Heaven are opened, and our Father bids
    me come
From this silence so unbroken by the tread of human feet,
Over where immortal footsteps echo on the golden street,
Then, till then, dear Father, teach me, that through all these
    fearful depths,
In the silence that surrounds me, Thou art guiding still my
    steps;
And when life for me is over, even in Heaven may I once more
Hear again the sound of footsteps, my own footsteps on the
    floor?

PITTSFIELD, MASS.,
VALLEY FARM, *June* 22, 1880.

MY DEAR CARRIE :—I consider it a privilege to
give, what you have asked, the story of my re-
lease from bondage in answer to the "prayer of
faith " ; bondage that was dark, deep and mysterious, and of eighteen years' duration. Two months
previous to my twelfth birthday, I was taken sick
at school, with what shortly proved to be an attack
of measles. I was not dangerously ill, and as soon
as could be expected, I was about the house, apparently my former healthy, happy self. But the
first ride I attempted after the illness, brought on
a sort of nervous spasm, of short duration, but
sufficiently different from anything I had ever experienced before, to prove that all was not well.
For six months I was able to take long walks, eat
and sleep well, but steadily creeping upon me I
felt those strange inexplicable nervous feelings,
that changed life, and my desires concerning it.
During the following two years I had severe sick
spells, from which I would rally, after awhile, with
strong holds upon hope, but, at length, so thoroughly had disease overpowered me, I was obliged
to succumb, and awful suffering and depression it

was my lot to bear. Shortly after my removal
here, began a contest between sickness and health,
life and death, which it is neither pleasant, nor
profitable, to attempt to describe.

What I have suffered, hoped, and feared, it is
beyond my power to tell. Many physicians have
attended my case, but although, in some instances,
temporary relief has been obtained, nothing permanent has been granted, except the knowledge that,
in my case, "vain is the help of man."

After the summer of 1867 I was confined wholly
to the house and mostly to my bed, being, very
frequently, for days at a time, utterly unable to
lift my head from the pillow, or be moved the
least particle without agony. During the summer
of 1868, under the careful treatment of Dr. A. M.
Smith, of this city, I was much relieved of spinal
and nervous trouble, and shall never cease thanking God for timely aid afforded ; for several subsequent years, under this physician's care, had more
comfortable times allotted me than I had known
for a long period of time before, but a sufferer I
was still, and must have remained, had not the
dear Master graciously interposed in my behalf.

I was unable to walk or stand *one moment* alone

upon my feet, a terrible dizziness, and pressure in the heart, attending every attempt of this kind. The cords of my lower limbs were contracted. For sixteen years I had not been able to lie an instant upon my left side; could take but small quantities of food, and often, for weeks at a time, was unable to take the least nourishment without great increase of pain. In one of your letters you speak of what you suffered from " exaltation of sensibility." How much that means to me ! During seasons of great prostration I have lain, for hours at a time, in that condition that had a person entered my room, had there been any unusual noise (how I used to pray that nothing of the kind might occur), I do not know how I could have endured it. My dear mother used to sit in the room adjoining mine, doing all in her power to hinder increase of excitement. I have endured the most excruciating pain, and have suffered about as much, it seems to me, as poor humanity could endure.

How zealously I strove to overcome disease, and regain my health, willing to submit to the most severe experiments suggested by physicians, if offered thereby any hope of relief, many can testify.

Last July, and once more in September, prayer was offered for me by Dr. Charles Cullis, of Boston, Mass. I was blessed spiritually, but was not yet prepared to take hold upon the promises, and claim a physical cure. About this time I was led to plead for a consecrated heart, and began to taste the blessedness of giving myself wholly away to God; began to ask, and receive, answers to my prayers in so remarkable a manner, that I could doubt no longer the willingness of Jehovah to *speak to the children of men.*

At some future time, I want to give you the particulars concerning special answers to prayer in a time of great wonderment and depression in regard to financial embarrassments.

Very soon reports were brought me concerning the great faith of some colored people of Wolcott-ville, Conn. (your own case, my dear Carrie, being prominent among those that helped increase my courage), and as these good people were soon expecting to visit Pittsfield, I was advised to see them. But alas! like Naaman, I questioned whether the waters of Israel were any better than those of Pharpar and Abana; why my own prayers, or those of my Christian neighbors,

might not avail as much as the prayers of Mrs.
Mix. I think one of the most important truths
which I have been called to learn, since coming to
this life of faith, is, that of all His children the
Lord demands obedience.

Looking unto Him, prayerfully, I was led to
Mrs. Mix. On the second of November she came
to me, prayed with me—friends in various parts of
the house uniting in prayer for me at the same
time—and without assistance from any human
agency, *I arose and walked;* no dizziness seized
me, nor was there any inclination to fall. I had
said in the morning that if, in this life, I was *ever*
able to walk to mother's kitchen and, coming
through certain rooms, back to my bed, I would
say I was *healed.*

Before dark, on that long to be remembered
Sunday, I accomplished this feat easily, and mother
and daughter praised God from fervent hearts.
Cords so long contracted *straightened in one
night.* I could now take food regularly without
distress, and the word of the Master came to me
with power : " Wait on the Lord : be of good
courage, and He shall strengthen thine heart;
wait, I say, on the Lord."—Psalm xxvii. 14.

I had yet to learn many lessons, however; among other things, that what I had now commenced is termed, and is, in truth, the very "*fight* of faith." I think I have met every foe that Pilgrim encountered on the first part of his journey from the city of Destruction, from Worldly Wiseman down to Simple and Presumption; each has had his say. Thanks be to God, I am trusting still.

Not many days had passed before old symptoms returned, and, according to human appearances, there was *need* of medicine. The tempter began an argument with my soul, somewhat difficult to resist, telling me that I could go no further without this, which had been my help so many years. In an agony of suspense and fear I came direct to God for light, for direction; and He spoke peace to my soul. I gave orders for my medicine to be thrown away; whether I could lift my head or not, I would trust !

Among other inestimable blessings, my Lord has granted me a mother strong in faith; when my own began to waver, hers but shone the clearer, and together we fought on. On the third of November, walking a short distance from our door, I had plucked a green leaf and borne it triumphantly to mother, by whom it was received as truly an evidence that the waters were abating, as was the olive leaf by Noah. I gained so rapidly, that, in the course of a few weeks, taking a friend's arm and a cane, I walked across the street to sister's.

O, it is all too glorious to describe, the wondrous way my Lord has led me on, seeming sometimes " for a small moment " to have forsaken me, but with " everlasting mercy " bearing me in mind. Gradually (my first word from the dear Lord, when I came to Him for healing, had been " wait ") my faith and strength increased, until I could walk some little distance on the frozen earth each day, and make short calls at near neighbors. We had lived in our house for seventeen years, and never, until since my cure, had I seen the upper rooms. Each trip upstairs seemed as new, and grand, and strange, as most people's trips to Europe.

Meanwhile, matters had been so arranged that the coming spring, my only sister was expecting to move one mile away, and was very desirous of taking mother and myself with her to her new home; but above everything, this side of death, stood my *dread of riding*. For eighteen years every attempt to ride had occasioned *spasms*, followed by such long prostration as was terrible to recall, and just here Satan stood over me exultant for many days.

I did not always wisely remember that God's Word does not promise aid in advance of trial, but " *as thy day* so shall thy strength be." When the full time for my first experience in the carriage came, the recollection of the agony I had endured in times past, for a moment overpowered me; my strength left me, my heart grew tremulous, and I called mightily unto God for help, for some word of cheer. Opening the good Book, expectantly, I was directed to these words : " He giveth power to the faint, and to them that have no might He increaseth strength."—Isaiah xl. 29. What could I ask more.

I went to the carriage, praising God. Victory did not crown my first effort, nor the next, but knowing that my Lord had promised—victory *must be mine.* All in good time it came; no larger than the cloud for which Elijah waited, was its first appearance, but by degrees I found that I could bear the motion of the carriage, and still better as time went on. I could be drawn slowly across the yard, but the thought of that one-mile drive terminating in change of home and surroundings, which I was so soon expected to undertake, Satan was permitted to hold before my mind's eyes for many days and nights, harassing me with doubts and fears, terrible to endure. On the twentieth of May, in an easy carriage phaeton, drawn by a gentle horse, I rode a quarter of a mile without spasms or any great distress. Victory was mine; friends stood upon the sidewalk, speaking words of encouragement and praise as we passed along, and the thankfulness that went up from my heart that afternoon, no one but the dear Master knows anything about.

Now I began coming to the dear Lord for unwavering faith concerning that long-dreaded removal to my new home, and on the morning of the second of June, little dreaming that that was the day appointed by the dear Master for the same, my cry unto him was answered by these words of promise, "Behold I am with thee, and will keep thee in all places whither thou goest * * * for I will not leave thee until I have done that which I have spoken to thee of."—Gen. xxviii. 15.

There had been no time appointed for my transit to other quarters, but that June morning it was as if my Lord had told me that the time was near at hand. To my great amazement, nervous anxiety was removed. I was wonderfully at rest, and began making preparations for a hasty exit; whether that day, or three months from that day, none but the dear Lord knew.

During the early part of the afternoon I was enabled to call at a certain neighbor's, whom I had desired to visit before leaving our old home, and make a farewell call at another place not far away. Returning home, somewhat exhausted, I sought my bed for rest, and rest was granted. And now, at the *right moment*, my brother-in-law, at his store some little distance away, whom I had not seen for some time, and to whom no one had spoken of calling for me to ride that day, was impressed to come to us with horse and phaeton. The time was now fully come. I was gloriously strengthened; rode to my new home without injury, or any great fatigue. Was not my Lord fulfilling His word of promise, gloriously? Is it any wonder if my soul is so filled with praise that the one hundred and third Psalm will keep surging up from its very depths? I have given you a somewhat lengthy account, but the story can never be half told. I am in a delightful place to praise God all the day long, am growing stronger and better as the days go by, have long since lain on my left side; in short, am being made *every whit whole,* thanks be to God, Who " giveth us the victory through our Lord Jesus Christ."

ALICE M. BALL.

GOODRICH, GENESEE Co., MICH., June, 1880.

DEAR FRIEND:—Some time since I solicited your prayers for my daughter; now I write to tell that we feel without a doubt she is cured. Oh, what a wonderful thing this faith cure is, for we can take hold of the promises of God with an unyielding grasp, and expect answers to our prayers. I feel that my faith is stronger now than it ever was before, and how we thank you that you united with us in prayer for her recovery; now we don't pray for her to be healed, but we thank God every day that he has cured her. I hope this faith cure may go on until thousands are cured; now, as I close, let me thank you again, and thank God for what he has done for us, with regards to you.

MRS. N. H. FARR.

GOODRICH, MICH., June 22.

DEAR FRIEND:—Though a stranger, a dear friend, I can of a truth testify to the words of my mother, and would feel condemned a great sinner before God, if, when I kneel to pray, I would not thank him for his blessings towards me. Now, Mrs. Mix, accept my thanks for your prayers, as I feel it has been a cure and a lesson of faith to me; kind regards to you, Mrs. Mix, and if it should be convenient, and you would not find it a burden, write to me.

Yours truly,

ELNORA I. FARR.

————

BURRVILLE, August 23, 1880.

I have been requested to give to the public an account of what has been done for me within the past two years, and perhaps some suffering one may see it and feel encouraged, and accept the way laid down in the word of God to be healed by faith. I cannot tell you much of the thirty-four years of my life that I have spent an invalid, shut out from the world and confined to a sick room; those years were filled up with disappointments, self-denial, and very much suffering. I was not twenty-one when I became an invalid; I think I had spinal disease, with acute inflammation of the kidneys.

At the commencement of my sickness, I seemed to lose all muscular power; I could not raise myself in bed, or get out of my chair alone; could not raise my feet upon the lower round of a chair for several years. I soon began to show that I was full of scrofula, and as I advanced in years other diseases and weaknesses came, and all that medicine or the skill of physicians could do, did not bring me health or the muscular power that I so much needed; medicine relieved for a little time, but did not cure. My case seemed mysterious and very difficult to understand, and I lived along in this miserable, sickly way, thirty-four years, and I concluded to wait patiently God's time and accept whatever came. But I really had no expectation in life. I had spells of hemorrhage twelve years, and was often brought so low that I could not speak aloud for three weeks, and my physician could find no pulse for a week, and one time I lay one hundred and twenty days without being able to sit up long enough to eat one meal. I had to lie in one position for several months at a time. I have not lain an hour upon my left side for twelve years because of a heart difficulty. I have had dropsy by spells for fifteen years, and became a monstrous body; my natural weight was not one hundred pounds, but I looked as if I would weigh nearly two hundred, and my dresses measured around the waist one yard and three-quarters. My limbs below the knee had become small, had been perishing for two years; there seemed scarcely any circulation in them; they appeared to be more dead than alive. About four years ago a gravelly substance began to work out of my flesh about the size of small pin heads, coming through the pores of the skin, and are found in all the scrofula sores I have, and I have had two hundred of them at one time, and I think it would be safe to say there has full eight quarts of this mysterious substance worked out of my flesh up to the present time. My family physician is a man of many years' experience; he said he never saw anything like it, and would not have believed it if he had not seen it himself; and in connection with this I would say that very many large gravel stones have formed in the kidneys, giving me terrible distress, such as I never can express.

In the fall of 1878 I heard of the cures that Mrs. Mix of Wolcottville had performed; at that time I was going down fast, and I felt that I could not live long. I heard that she had been instrumental in restoring the sight of a blind woman in Wolcottville, and I thought if she could restore sight to the blind and make the lame to walk, perhaps there could be something done for me. I had been impressed more than a year that medicine would never cure me, and nothing but an Almighty power could do it, and I must trust in the Lord for it. The most that I could walk for years was from two to three yards, holding up by everything that came in my way. Mrs. Mix was sought for, and she came to see me November 7, 1878. She came full of faith, believing the Lord would raise me up and restore me to health, and after the first treatment I walked out of my bed-room, across the sitting-room and back, and from that time there was a change. I had power to walk given me, although my feet and limbs seemed so nearly dead. I had a great deal to contend with; my whole body was diseased, and since that time have been walking about the house and out of doors. I first began to walk in November,

and the next May was the first time I put my feet
upon the ground in twenty-four years; everything
around looked to me like a new creation. I could
then praise God and take courage; my heart was
full of thanksgiving and praise. The change was
very gradual; in about four days after Mrs. Mix's
first visit I had a severe sick spell; it was not like
anything I experienced in all the thirty-four years
of my sickness. But it was evident there was a
change taking place to throw off disease. It is
now some more than a year and a half since I
began to get better, and in that time I have had
ten of those spells, and they are all attended with
dropsy. I am much less in size after each one,
and find I am better than before; in one of those
sick spells I lay in a sweat five days. I am very
much reduced in size, and am looking quite like
other people. My right lung had been inactive,
and I think I had no use of it for years, and it was
evident the lung was diseased. I believed there
was an abscess or some sort of a sore in the lower
part of the lung. I became very sick from the
lung disease. But in a few days I felt that it was
restored and just as well as the other, only somewhat weaker, and at the present time feel no pain

or difficulty about it. I am not strong and well yet, but I am changing all the time for the better. I walk about the yard and go about the house and do light work, feeling that I must use the strength God has given to some purpose, and I so much enjoy going about from room to room, although it seems strange to hear the sound of my own footsteps after being shut away in my room so many years. It is beautiful to me to look back and see what care the Lord has taken of me for a year and a half. I have not taken a spoonful of medicine in that time, although I have had ten severe sick spells. I have trusted in the Lord to raise me up and he has brought me safe through every time. I feel there must have been a *divine agency* in all this, or I should have died. I believe it is of the Lord. Oh, I have had such joy and peace in trusting in our Heavenly Father. I am learning to trust in Him for everything. This living by faith gives spiritual life and joy and comfort, such as we can obtain from no other source. I am not perfectly well and strong, but I am trusting in the Lord for a full restoration of health and strength in His own good time.

MRS. SARAH M. BURR.

"HAVE FAITH IN GOD."

No. 260 Connecticut Street,
Buffalo, N. Y., July 7, 1880.

On the sixth of January, 1877, after a gradual decline in health, I was prostrated with an attack of fever, proceeding from my spine, the result, probably, of a severe fall on a stone sidewalk several months before. The fever was soon subdued, but my disease grew into settled spinal difficulty, and from the inflammation of the spinal nerves proceeded a most distressing hyper-acuteness, called hyperæsthesia. This extended to all my large joints; and my hips, knees and ankles could not be touched even by myself, on account of their sensitiveness. The disease increased until the nerves in the joints were so unnaturally alive that it was as if they had been laid bare, and it seemed to me as though nothing less than spasms would be the immediate result were they touched. The vibrating of these sensitive nerves, occasioned by the tiniest jar or noise in the room, was something indescribably dreadful.

For all but the first two months of my illness, extreme helplessness as well as suffering made my lot almost unendurable. For more than two years, turning over alone or moving myself a particle in bed was simply an impossibility. Every move was made for me with the greatest care. I suffered intensely with my head; the violent, tearing pain, the terrible sense of weight, and the extreme sensitiveness made a soft, small pillow feel like a block of stone, the pressure of which was crushing my brain to atoms. Much of the time we were obliged to exclude from the room all excepting those who had the care of me.

For eleven months I could not sit up at all, but in the spring of 1878 improved slowly, and could be lifted into a chair for a little while each day. I was more comfortable until July, but I could not by my greatest exertions get able to help myself at all. The only way in which I could be moved from the bed to the chair, was by being lifted under my arms, as I could endure no pressure on my spine.

The very warm weather at that time, and my making attempts to help myself when in such a weak condition, caused a sudden and violent relapse, and, in spite of everything that could be done for me, I continued to fail. I rallied a little in the autumn, but only temporarily.

In January, 1879, my mother's mother, who had lived with us for years and who was very dear to me, died at our house, after a short illness. I was so low at the time that there could be no public notice of her death, and only a few intimate friends were admitted into our silent house.

By the middle of February, my weakness was so great that most of the time I could scarcely speak in a whisper, and sometimes could only move my lips. Often the exertion of whispering one word would cause the perspiration to start profusely; and I would lie for hours needing something rather than ask for it. I could take no solid food whatever, and it exhausted me greatly to swallow even liquid food.

My disease had grown into blood consumption; I was emaciated to a shadow, and my largest veins looked like mere threads. Nothing could keep me warm, and the chill of death seemed upon me. A great part of the time I lay gasping faintly for breath, and I suffered excruciatingly. Even the weight of my arms and limbs seemed to be almost unendurable, and this terrible strain was constant. My pulse could scarcely be found, and I was not expected to live from one day to the next. Dr.

Davis, a well known physician of Attica, tried his skill, but failed. Dr. Baethig of this city also treated the case with a like result. Then Dr. Lon See On, a Chinese physician, educated in his own country, was called. He is a gifted fellow, and treated the case, but was unable to do any good. Everything that the most skillful physicians could do for me had been done; only the "Great Physician" could restore me by His almighty power. I have no doubt that it was ordered by Providence, that, just at this time, there should appear in the daily paper a short account of the wonderful cures performed in answer to the prayers of Mrs. Edward Mix, a colored lady, of Wolcottville, Conn. The article represented her as an earnest, humble Christian, who simply professed to be doing God's work. She had herself been cured, after years of ill health, by the prayers and laying on of hands of a Rev. Mr. Allen, of Springfield. Mother mentioned these facts to me, and the more I thought on the subject, the more I felt that a letter must be written her in regard to my own case. I had often heard of faith cures before this, and there had been read to me some portions of W. W. Patton's book, "Remarkable Answers to Prayer," but, although not discrediting them, none had ever produced so great an impression on my mind as this short account of Mrs. Mix. I waited a few hours, then requested my sister to write her that I believed her great faith might avail for me, if she would pray for my recovery, even if she were not present to lay her hands upon me. On Tuesday, February 25th, her answer came as follows:

WOLCOTTVILLE, CONN., February 24, 1879.

MISS CARRIE JUDD:—I received a line from your sister Eva, stating your case, your disease and your faith. I can encourage you, by the Word of God, that, "according to your faith," so be it unto you; and besides you have this promise, "The prayer of faith shall save the sick, and the Lord shall raise him up." Whether the person is present or absent, if it is a "prayer of faith," it is all the same, and God has promised to raise up the sick ones, and if they have committed sins to forgive them. Now this promise is to you, as if you were the only person living. Now if you can claim that promise, I have not the least doubt but what you will be healed. You will first have to lay aside all medicine of every description. Use

no remedies of any kind for anything. Lay aside
trusting in the "arm of flesh," and lean wholly
upon God and His promises. When you receive
this letter I want you to begin to pray for faith,
and Wednesday afternoon the female prayer-meeting is at our house.* We will make you a subject
of prayer, between the hours of three and four. I
want you to pray for yourself, and pray believing,
and then *act faith*. It makes no difference how
you feel, but get right out of bed and begin to
walk by faith. Strength will come, disease will
depart and you will be made whole. We read in
the Gospel, "Thy faith hath made thee whole."
Write soon.   Yours in faith,

                              MRS. EDWARD MIX.

Is it any wonder that in my utter weakness, my
confirmed helplessness, and, above all, my lack of
faith, that I was tempted to smile unbelievingly
at the words, "get right out of bed and begin to
walk by faith"? My conscience reproved me for
my unbelief, and I began to pray for an increase
of faith. I left off all medicine at once, though I

---

* But the weather being stormy no one came, so there was
none to pray but Mr. Mix and myself.

confess it was with a struggle, for I was very dependent upon it for *temporary* alleviation of my extreme suffering. At the hour appointed by Mrs. Mix, members of our own family also offered up prayer, though not in my room. Just before this, I seemed to have no power, whatever, to grasp the promise. Terrible darkness and powerful temptations from Satan rose to obscure even the little faith I had, but suddenly my soul was filled with a childlike peace and confidence different from anything I had ever before experienced.

There was no excitement, but, without the least fear or hesitation, I turned over and raised up alone, for the first time in over two years. My nurse, Mrs. H., who had taken care of me for nearly a year, was greatly affected, and began praising God for His wonderful power and mercy.

Directly after, with a little support from my nurse, I walked a few steps to my chair. During that same hour, a decided change was perceptible in my color, circulation and pulse, and I could talk aloud with ease. Referring to my diary, which was kept by Mrs. H., I find under February 27th, which was the day after my restoration: "Carrie moved herself in bed several times during the night. This afternoon she walked from her chair to the bed, a distance of about eight feet, by taking hold of my arms. The Lord strengthens her every hour, both physically and in faith. Blessed be His holy Name! " Then, under February 28th: " Carrie grows stronger, moves herself more easily, rests better nights, has a good appetite. I gave her a sponge-bath this afternoon, and I could not but notice the change in the color of her flesh; instead of the yellow, dead look, it is pink and full of life." Under March 1st: "This morning she drew on her stockings." March 2d: "Her chest and lungs have been strong; she has talked aloud a great deal. Appetite good; color fresh and clear."

In about three weeks I could walk around the room without even having any one near me; in four weeks I walked down stairs with a little assistance; I walked very steadily from the first, and my joints, which had been so weakened by the hyperæsthesia, grew strong and firm at once. My muscles filled out very rapidly, but I suffered nothing from aching or lameness, even after I commenced going up and down stairs.

The first pleasant day in April I went out of

doors and into a neighbor's. It seemed as though it was almost too much joy to comprehend, to really be out in the air and sunshine once more. I looked up at the windows of my room with a vague idea that there must be imprisoned there still, a prostrate, suffering creature, of whom I had once been a part, but now was freed from by some mysterious process. The thought of my long and terrible suffering, and of my sudden and joyful deliverance, almost overwhelms me now as I review it all so minutely.

I will mention here, that it was especially noticeable, during my healing, that whenever I made any extra exertion of my own, suddenly, and without the least apparent cause, my strength would fail me. It was soon revealed to me, that I was simply to look to the Lord for improvement; that as He had begun the work, He would carry it on without any strivings on my part.

The more fully I cast myself upon Him, the more I was supported, and often I felt borne up as if by some buoyancy in the air, while there was little or no effort of my own. Even more wonderful, and infinitely more precious, than being brought from death unto life, physically, is the

renewed life which the soul experiences at the
same time under the healing influence of the Holy
Spirit. A deep, intense love for God is implanted
in the heart, worldly desires and ambitions sink
into nothingness, the one absorbing thought is to
be conformed more and more to the image of
Christ, and the forgiveness of sins promised with
the healing in James v. 14, 15, is experienced as
never before.

My gain in flesh and strength was rapid, and
my friends say that I am now looking better than
ever before. The trouble in my head, which was
almost constant for a long time before my prostration, entirely disappeared when I was cured,
and I can do a vast amount of studying and writing without even a slight headache. I can also
take very long walks and enjoy them.

All glory be to our merciful and loving Redeemer! and that I may ever abide in Him, and
bring forth the "fruit of the Spirit," is the daily
prayer of my life.

CARRIE F. JUDD.

With my kind pastor's permission I publish
the following letter; his reply to one which I received from a stranger:

No. 790 Seventh Street,
Buffalo, N. Y., March 13, 1880.

Dear Sir:—Miss Judd has shown me your favor of the 11th inst., and requests me to vouch for her entire credibility.

I do this with great pleasure, the more so that I have known her so long, and have been entirely conversant with all the facts in the case, from the beginning. I can assure you of her long and painful illness, of her utter and complete prostration, of the immediate expectation of death by herself and all her friends; during all those months I ministered at her bedside, and saw her draw nearer and nearer to the end.

But suddenly, and, of course, by the interposition of God, and doubtless in answer to the prayers of the Church and of the faithful, she was, so to speak, in a day restored, and is now in perfect health. Of these facts I assure you. They are well known to all here, and you have only to ask any resident of Buffalo to be satisfied of the truthfulness of all that she may tell you.

Why should it be accounted strange that God should raise one of his children from the bed of death? I confess I see no reason. His promise was for all time, "unto you, and to your children," and if we gain less now, it is because we are less faithful, and not because His promise is less sure.

I shall be glad to give you any further information in my power, if you desire it.

Very truly,   C. F. A. BIELBY,

Rector St. Mary's-Church-on-the-Hill (Episcopal).

WEST MERIDEN, August 19.

I was taken sick two years ago last spring with nervous prostration and sciatic rheumatism, which made me unable to walk. I have been confined to the house and to my bed most of the time. I had three different physicians, but did not seem to get any better. Last October I had a dreadful cough come on which made me much worse.

Mrs. Mix visited me last April; from that very hour I began to improve. I walked down stairs that evening, and the next day I rode out.

I am now so I can walk any ordinary distance. My cough has wholly left me.

Respectfully,

CARRIE B. RICE.

BURNHAM HOUSE, EAST BRIDGFORD,
NOTTINGHAMSHIRE, ENGLAND, February, 16, 1880.

DEAR MRS. MIX:—I am very, very much obliged
for your kind letters, and especially for an interest
in your prayers which I still much need. I am
still gaining strength in spite of the cold, stormy
weather, but it rather tries my chest.

I keep my eye upon my Great Physician, and
constantly take my pain and weakness to Him.
I can walk now two miles at once; it is a great
change. I saw my surgeon three weeks ago; he
said my restoration was a "perfect miracle." He
would as soon have thought of seeing his baby six
months old walk as me. It is such a blessing to
have such a precious physician to fly to in our
weakness.

I am far from strong yet. My complaints are
numerous. Three of my medical men have wished
me to undergo an operation for one complaint I
suffer from, but I keep laying it before the Lord
and expect Him to heal *completely*. I am sure He
is able and perfectly willing. My home is being
broken up in March, owing to the death of my
parents, which, of course, is very trying for me in
my weakness. There is a great deal to excite and

upset me. Do pray for the Lord to guide, instruct and keep me. I am so delicate that every one seems afraid to take me in. Yet the Lord I know will open some door and direct me.

I intend if the Lord strengthens me to recommence my work amongst the poor in Lincoln. Do ask the Lord to fit me, if He intends it. I long to win souls for Him. I have *nothing to live* for but *His glory.* I should have written before but have had so much to think of. I know you will like to hear how I am. I have thought of publishing my case of healing for God's glory and the encouragement of others. If you write to me before the last of March, address as before, please.

Believe me, yours sincerely, in Christ Jesus,
MISS LOUISE LOCKWOOD.

Mrs. E. Mix.   NEW HAVEN, June 30, 1880.

My Dear Friend:—I take pleasure in writing you the explanation of my case, and how wonderfully I am being healed through *faith* and *trust* in *God.*

I have been an invalid for seven years the middle of August, with scrofula, rheumatic inflammation of the throat, spine and nerves, and tubercles. When you first called to see me (a little over a year ago), I was very weak and extremely nervous, my spine and throat being a very agonizing trouble, having three weeks previous to your call a very ill turn. I had not my voice above a low whisper, and growing much worse daily, could not use my left arm of any account; my right one I could use to take my medicine when as well as usual. The pain was so acute in my spine I could hardly turn in bed at all; my lungs were also very sensitive, one of them the doctors called entirely diseased, troubled for breath, etc. My tonsils eaten out by ulceration, and that caused the epiglottis to enlarge about twice the natural size; this trouble had reached to the stomach and bowels, and often choked me, especially when I had the terrible paroxysm in the spine and throat, the effects often lasting ten days before I could feel very much relief in my spine. My bowels troubled me continually, with constipation. I had to be lifted in the most careful manner from my bed to an easy rocker once a week when able to have my bed made, then back again as quick as possible. I have not taken any medicine for the six months past, and not anything of any account since you first called to see me.

I enjoy your calls so much, for your strong faith encourages mine greatly to have you pray with and for me, anointing me with oil in the name of the Lord, believing that I may be healed if I will put perfect trust and confidence in Him who is able and willing to alleviate our sufferings. I did, and our prayers were answered in a great measure in about an hour after you left. I received strength in my spine and throat to be able to speak so I could be heard in the adjoining room. Then in twenty-four hours I could move my partially paralyzed limb, with considerable exertion, off the edge of the bed, but remember at that time I had not been able for three years to move my limbs of any account.

My second relief was to be able to walk with the aid of a cane and some one standing the other side of me, from my bed to an easy rocker in the middle of the room, which is about eight feet. The first time in trying to walk I could not place my heel down to the floor without falling backwards on account of the acute pain it caused in my spine. I tried to walk on my toes for several weeks so as to try and get my heel down. Then with my Heavenly Father's strength I became able to turn over in bed easily and look out of the window and do considerable crocheting. I could not read very much at this time. The next improvement, I could go from my bed to the next room (opposite side), to a lounge, and sit bolstered up an hour and a half twice a week with the aid of a cane and some one standing back of me to steady my spine if I reeled backwards, as I was liable to do, as I could not get my heel quite down to the floor. Then back to the bed again in the same manner. You may think it strange when I tell you I could go back to bed even better than I went from it. You may ask what was the reason? It was answer to fervent prayer to God while sitting up. He helped me to lean on Him with more confidence, and my lame limb would go down to the floor easier.

The next improvement which God saw best to give me was to drop my cane and trust more fully in His strength. Now I am able to go into the other room alone (some one being near me). The Lord said, "As thy days are, so shall thy strength be;" and "All thing are possible to him that believeth." These and many others are precious promises to me. I am improving every day in some respect, but the hot weather does not give me quite as much strength as the cooler days. My case has changed since there was so much improvement in my lungs, for I used to like the warmer days the best, but now the cooler ones are preferable. My bowels are in better condition. It is as you have told me, that my nerves will be the last thing to be healed, for when I become stronger my nerves will receive more real strength, and at last I hope I shall come off conqueror, with the "Divine Power" aiding me. I have not the least doubt but that He has something yet in store for me to do. My earnest plea is what He will have me to do, and that I may have strength given me to do it to His honor and glory. God does answer prayer in the most wonderful ways. He has given us the power to help in this missionary work, by giving me strength to take my pencil and write to my friends, or our prayers in silent but faithful effort to do His will in everything as far as He gives us strength. Oh, how sure and precious are His promises.

The last improvement, thus far, I have been

permitted with strength to ride out twice, an hour at a time. In whatever way the Lord has seen best to improve my health, it has seemed to be lasting; my limb has not gone back, neither has my voice, but is being strengthened continually; am now sitting bolstered up one hour and a half, to two hours at a time, which is not gaining quite as fast as some, but God does not think best that I should get right up as He permits others to do. I am thankful for a little improvement for the better if it does seem slow; there are a great many chronic difficulties to contend with; as the doctors used to say, your case is a peculiar one; it takes time for some to be healed, while others are getting well in an instant as it were, by the power of God and answer to the prayer of faith. It was a long time before I thought I should have to give up to sickness, but when the time came it was sudden, and I think I shall be healed sudden at last, just as soon as the dear Lord sees best to take away all disease and give me entire strength I am waiting His own best time. I am now so I can read a little more at a time, and remember what I read better than any time during my long illness. I consider this a great blessing. It used to be like

a hammer beating on my brain to read, or have
much read to me. I thank you, Mrs. Mix, for the
many earnest prayers you have offered in my behalf, and for the answer God has been so kind
to give me. My prayer. is that you may long
live to be the instrument of much good in this
world, through the power of " Our Divine Master."
I hope the time will soon come when all invalids
cannot say I am sick, but that God has washed me
with His blood and made me whole. I think that
" Each promise is a staff if we have faith to lean
on it; God is wiser than man; let Him rule." To
Him I give the praise for my restoration to health
thus far. You may use all or part of this as you
think best, for the " Glory of God."

On the 25th day of July, I was able to be carried in an easy chair by boat and baggage car to
Ocean Grove, and by the blessing of the Lord I
was soon able to go to Miss Jennie Smith's home
in Burlington, N. J. This dear sister was healed
in answer to believing prayer after sixteen years
of utter helplessness. October 6th I arrived at
my home in New Haven to the surprise of my
neighbors and friends, and when Sabbath came I
walked to church, where I had not been for over

eight years, and I can say, let all the earth praise the Lord.

Jennie Smith has been telling the Green street Methodist congregation, Philadelphia, that she was cured of a chronic spinal disease by a miracle. She was bedridden for sixteen years. A few months ago, when she was in the Homœopathic Hospital, she asked Dr. John C. Morgan to pray with her, as she felt that she was going to sit up. He did so, and in a few minutes afterward she sat up in her chair. This was after all trials to bolster her up by means of pillows and hands had failed. From this time she began to have a strong belief that she would be able to walk again, and at length she appointed a certain time for a miraculous cure. Some of her friends were invited. To others she wrote asking them to offer up specific prayer on her behalf on that day. After waiting until nearly midnight she asked two persons present to take her by the arms, as she felt that the time had come. They complied, and, with barely any effort on their part, she rose to her feet and walked. Since that time she has had complete use of her limbs. Dr. Morgan declares the truth of her story.

From your friend, trusting in Jesus,

M. E. HALL.

DAMASCUS, April 27, 1881.

You wished me to write something concerning my sickness and my recovery by prayer. I will try to do so. For a number of years preceding my sickness, I seemed to be gradually failing in health, each year growing weaker and weaker, until April 1st, 1879, I was suddenly prostrated with heart disease, the physicians said ; and for twenty months I could not stand upon my feet, or sit up, and most of the time could not raise my head from my pillow. More than half of the time I seemed to be hovering between life and death. I suffered as it seems death itself. My nerves were so sensitive, that it was almost impossible to endure the slightest sound. With my other diseases I began bloating with dropsy. It soon settled round my heart. The water round the heart caused those awful sinking spells, that I cannot describe, nor do I wish to, for I do not like to think of them. I was getting discouraged, for I knew that I could not live much longer, and through all my sickness I had a strong desire to get well, although I did not say much about it. Then a friend heard of Mrs. Mix, and wrote to her concerning me. She sent her reply to me, saying that she would pray for me on the 17th of November, and that I must pray for faith and strength to be given me, and that I might be restored to health. It seemed rather strange to me at first, but as I thought more about it, it became plainer, and I thought that I would try. I commenced praying for faith, and when the hour came and my friends arrived, who were to offer up prayer in my behalf, I was not excited in the least. While they were praying I was alone in my room, which was my wish, and when they had ceased praying I sat up in bed, something I could not do before without great trouble with my heart. Then they put me in the rocking-chair, and I sat there a few minutes. My friends came in to see me sitting up, a sight they never expected to witness. While sitting up I requested another prayer, which was granted, and we thanked and praised the Lord together. I tried sitting up every day for a week; then I caught a heavy cold which sent the water around my heart again, and for three weeks I was very sick. On the 15th of December, 1880, Mrs. Mix was praying for a neighbor, who had been bedridden for years. I knew of it and was praying for him too, though I

was feeling very badly myself. I was trying to
eat a little dinner, but my appetite was so poor
that I could not eat anything. Suddenly I felt as
if I could sit up, so they helped me up on the side
of the bed. Then I wanted to stand on my feet.
They put me on my feet, and assisted me to
walk a few steps; then I said, let me go, and
I walked all round the room. I went out in
the kitchen, which is quite a distance. I came
back to my own room and took my singing-
book and sung piece after piece just as loud and
clear as I ever sang. Oh, I was so happy, I did
not know what I said or did. In a few minutes I
wanted to take a ride. The horse and cutter were
brought, and I walked out on the porch and down
the steps to the cutter without much assistance.
I took a short ride; I did not go to bed again that
day; I have been gaining ever since; I have been
to church twice. How good it seemed to be there
again. The distance to the church is about five
miles; I did not come back the same day. I ride
out almost every day. I can walk all round the
house on the first floor, and have walked a little
distance on the ground several times. When I
get very tired my heart troubles me some, but the

Lord has done much for me, and can do much
more. "The Lord is nigh unto all them that call
upon Him." I have felt the loving presence of
Jesus more than I ever did before. I will ask you
to remember me in your faith meetings, that I may
be entirely restored to health, and that I may trust
always in Jesus, who has done so much for me.

L. D. TYLER.

This lady fully recovered and was married one
year from the day she was first prayed for.

ADAMS NERVINE ASYLUM,
JAMAICA PLAIN, MASS., August, 1881.

MRS. MIX :—For many years I have been an
invalid; for years together utterly helpless, at
other times able to walk from room to room, but
suffered intensely all this time. I came here January 1st, and have been confined to my bed since.
Several of the doctors here (there is only one exception) think I have *incurable* spine and other
diseases, and I am to leave here soon. I can step
a few steps, and only that. For years I have been
much interested in "prayer cures," and I have
been peculiarly led all these years.

Over a year ago (I had heard indirectly of you
before) I heard of one who was going to write

you to come to their home; then I thought it is
so near she can come to mine; but they changed
their minds. I sent to them for your address;
they thought they had lost it, etc., etc., and in no
way could I get it. Now I know it was God that
prevented it, as I was not quite ready for it.

Month by month, and even hour by hour, I have
been gradually led up to the present light, to
understand more fully the life of faith, and gradually as I could bear it, letters and leaflets have
come to me, and four days ago "The Prayer of
Faith," by Carrie F. Judd, came to me with wonderful help and strength, and although I had not
thought to write you till I left here, God has
spoken to me to write to you. For some reason
it has been very much harder even than usual to
write this; a hand seems holding mine firmly to
prevent my writing, and still God says, write, and
I try to obey His will. I shall make no excuses for
writing, for this *resistance* is something I do not
understand. I am surrounded by loving Christian
people, but none seem to have faith in prayer
cures, and that has tried my faith. One patient
who can come into my room occasionally is interested with me. She is one of God's noblest

women. She feels as do I, that we are so earnest that God must make known His will to us in some way. Sometimes we cannot meet, but we each pray in our own rooms for the other. Now is one of those times, but I cannot write you without mentioning her name too, Miss Carrie L. French, although she does not know. Will you pray for us? About *acting faith*, I would not be allowed to do more than at present, unless I say my pain is gone, or greatly relieved. I do feel it would be to God's glory to cure me suddenly, and show His power while I am here; but if He sees not best, or if he wishes to cure me gradually (I feel for one week I have been gaining and have slept three nights in answer to prayer), then His will be done. Please pray that *our* faith fail not, and that we may know His will, and if it is for His glory and honor we may be cured suddenly.

One lady who has done a noble missionary work, a lovely Christian, is despondent because she feels it wrong not to have faith.

One of the head managers, or rather superiors, said to her, "I cannot have faith in these faith cures, but if you, Miss Bowen, should be cured *now*, or Miss Cowles, I should have faith."

I would love dearly to be cured if it is *His will*, but I shall have strength to wait His time, here or in Heaven. O, if we only could have strength to receive the promises, it seems as if His name would be so glorified, especially in Miss Bowen's case. O, will you not as *soon as you receive this pray earnestly for us?* I think we are ready for the blessing so long denied till we were ready. Christ is very near us, and I *know* He told me to write to you, although it has been such a difficult task; how difficult only He knows who constantly told me I was doing His will, although it takes my utmost strength, and my back is so weak.

I beg of you, in the name of Christ, to help us.

If this reaches you so that you can answer before the 17th, or so it can reach here the night of the 19th, please direct as the heading of the letter. If not please enclose in another envelope, directed to Benj. S. Codman, M. D., 13 and 15 Tremont Street, Boston, Mass., and he will send it wherever I am. This is a delightful *Institute for nervous (not insane) people.* Mine is spinal trouble.

I fear there will be trouble in reading this, but that I cannot help, but God can.

I am one of Christ's little suffering ones.

ALMENA J. COWLES.

BOSTON, September 7, 1881.

MRS. MIX :—Your kind letter was received yesterday. The 24th of August I came here from the Nervine Asylum for a few days until the doctors could complete the arrangements to take me to " The Home for Incurables," in Brooklyn. I am now admitted, but shall not need to go, as at my request Dr. Peck, Miss Hawes, and my kind doctor, came to pray with me, August 30th, and I was healed by the dear Lord, after being anointed in His name by Dr. Peck, and I am gaining in strength every day; am dressed all day, and go up and down stairs several times in a day. I shall probably soon go to my home in or near Amherst, Mass. It is indeed a miracle, and I know that you will praise the Lord with me for His wonderful spiritual and physical blessing. Believe me *very, very* grateful for your kind letter. May the Lord bless you in the noble work to which He has called - you. For some reason it still tires me to write, and as I am situated cannot conveniently write with pen and ink, therefore you will pardon this.

Very respectfully and gratefully,

ALMENA J. COWLES.

63

ERIE, 3, 7, 1882.

SISTER MIX :—Beloved in the Lord. It gives
me pleasure to comply with your request in rela-
tion to my healing.

Taught from childhood to believe that the gift of
healing perished with the close of the Apostolic age,
I was slow to embrace the teachings of the Bible.

My malady had been from childhood, very seldom a day passed that I did not suffer more or
less with pain across my forehead, often so severe
as wholly to unfit me for the care of children or
household duties. In consequence of the intense
pain my eyesight was impaired, so that I had to
use glasses at twenty-five years of age. Vomiting
would sometimes afford me temporary relief, only
to be followed by more intense suffering ; so the
years passed by. My husband being a physician,
administered the usual remedies, indeed, everything available, with but transient benefit, so I
made up my mind to endure it to the end of life.

The gastric disturbance which often attended
the acute paroxysms of pain were of so intense a
character that the retching and vomiting would
only cease when my strength was so far exhausted
that I could no longer make the effort.

All this I suffered for thirty years ! In the fall of 1881 my attention was aroused to healing by prayer on reading Miss Judd's book. Sometime in December, 1881, my husband wrote you, requesting you to pray for my healing. I did not know he had done so until he received your answer, telling us to unite with you in prayer for healing on the first Wednesday in January, at 2.30 o'clock, P.M. We fasted on that day and offered earnest prayer for deliverance.

On the receipt of your letter, as stated above, I immediately laid aside all remedial agents, and committed my case wholly to God.

On Wednesday afternoon I realized great relief, " I saw men as trees walking," but on Thursday morning, blessed be God, the pain was gone, nor has it or the gastric disturbance returned. O, I have passed into a new world. Draw near, all ye of like precious faith, and unite with me in praise to my Redeemer, who hath done such great things for me.

My sleep is as peaceful and sweet as a child's, my head clear, appetite good, blessed be God, I am well.

Many thanks to you for the interest you have

taken in my welfare, the Lord reward you an hundred fold, and make you a blessing to many.

In the faith, respectfully,

MRS. DR. J. A. BASSETT.

NO. 99 GOFFE STREET,
NEW HAVEN, CONN., JUNE 29, 1880.

This is to certify that I, Leonard S. Turner, was taken very ill about November 29th, 1878, with hemorrhage of the lungs, and was confined to my bed until April, and had had the best of medical advice, and those physicians thinking my case a hopeless and incurable one, so at the last extremity, when breath appeared to be leaving the body, my family thought it advisable to consult with Mrs. Mix and husband, as she had been so highly recommended for her wonderful cures, that they sent for her, and by their joint supervision, under the instrumentality and faith in God, I was able to walk about the room in about one-half or three-quarters of an hour after their entrance. I am now able to attend to my business, and have not had to procure a physician since, simply by faith in prayer.

LEONARD S. TURNER.

KILLINGWORTH, CONN., December 9, 1881.

It is with pleasure that I give my testimony in regard to faith healing in the year of 1881. My eyes began troubling me, when suddenly they became so painful I was obliged to give up using them entirely. I consulted a skillful oculist. He said my eyes were in a very bad condition, and if I did not get help there was great danger of my getting entirely blind; after examining them closely he prescribed for me. I followed his directions, suitable glasses were procured, but the improvement was very slow, and in the month of May they became worse. I again went to the oculist to seek advice, hoping to obtain relief; after a space of time I felt a slight improvement, but in the month of June they were much worse. After the 20th of June I could not go out doors when the sun was shining, the pain in them was so severe it was impossible for me to bear the sunlight or lamplight. I was obliged to keep them bandaged, or stay in a dark room, that being the only way of relief from suffering. I was fully satisfied that the remedies used were not accomplishing the work. I had heard of faith cures for some time, and I verily believed in them, because I knew God's promises were true, I at once came to the conclusion that my eyes could be healed by faith in God. I knew the camp-meeting was to be held at Tylerville, the 20th of August, I was quite sure Mrs. Mix would be there; I resolved to see her and be healed. On the evening of the 24th I went to the camp ground and found Mrs. Mix's tent; after talking with her a few minutes I had perfect faith that I should be healed. She told me I must lay aside all medicine, and my glasses, and trust wholly in God's power for healing. I had worn glasses constantly for seven months or kept in a dark room, as the oculist had directed; unless I had believed that God would heal them then and there, in answer to prayer, nothing would have tempted me to have left off my glasses; but I believed and I took them off once for all. After we had prayed together Mrs. Mix anointed my eyes, and laid her hands on them in the name of Jesus, I left the tent believing I was healed. When I returned to a room where there was a light I felt none of the former pain in my eyes. On the 26th I again attended the camp-meeting, a ride of six miles, believing I should receive strength from God to do it, and I did, bless His holy name! On Sunday, the 28th, I went again in spite of the intense heat of the sun. I could see that I was gaining fast. Sometimes temptations came and my eyes felt a little weak. I would say: I am healed, and I will act faith; and so on I went trusting, I was confident the power that removed the pain would help me bear the trial. It is now over three months since I was healed, and my eyes are gaining rapidly every day. I use them several hours a day in sewing or reading, and I can do it without fear by simply trusting in God. I am more fully persuaded than ever before that all things are possible to him that believeth; the light of God's spirit is poured into my heart, and I am so happy trusting in the Lord.

> It is not for merit that I have done,
> It is not by effort of my own;
> But through His wondrous grace alone,
> I am kept by the power of God.

Yours in faith,

MISS ROSE NETTLETON.

I have written this testimony by lamp-light.

January 23, 1882.

DEAR MRS. MIX :—Because I have not been
miraculously raised from a *sick bed,* as have so many,
I have hesitated about giving my testimony to
the public; but when I look back upon the past
two years and see how wonderfully my life and
health have been preserved, in answer to believing
prayer, I feel that even my experience may be a
help to some other trembling one.

I had been an invalid the greater part of eighteen years, sometimes shut in my room for months,
then again strong enough to ride and do some
light work. Twice during this time I was quite
well for a year or more. One year and a half
before I was healed, I was suddenly taken *very ill.*
I did not leave the house for nearly a year. I was
able to ride, do some light work, and attend
church a few times during the summer, gaining
very slowly, suffering *much* from weakness and
nervous prostration.

As Mrs. Mix was in town about this time,
friends advised my seeing her. I called upon her
the evening of November 1st, with little expectation of receiving benefit.

After conversing with Mrs. Mix a few moments

upon the subject of faith and physical healing, she asked me to pray that I might be healed. I was at once forcibly impressed with the fact that I had never offered such a prayer, although an invalid so *many years*. I had asked God for patience and submission to His will, never thinking the prayer of faith could heal the sick.

After we had knelt in prayer Mrs. Mix anointed with oil in the name of the Lord, and soon asked if I thought I was healed. I acknowledged that I felt *no change,* no relief from pain. Mrs. Mix again knelt in prayer, and the *power of God then* possessed my entire being; all pain left me. I believed that I was healed, and said to those awaiting their turn in an adjoining room as I passed out, "I am healed, and in the name of the Lord expect to walk to church to-morrow." (I was stopping at grandparents' about quarter of a mile from church.) The change was so great I could but praise the Lord, when I awoke to consciousness during the night. The next morning I walked to church, attended Love Feast at nine o'clock, remained through morning service and Sunday school, rode two and a half miles to my home. I sat up through the afternoon, and at night felt very little fatigue. The following morning some of the old pain returned, and as I took my bed I began to wonder if I was really healed. I then remembered that I was to pray in the name of the Lord that this pain might be removed (St. Matt. xxi. 22.) While in prayer the same power came over me that I experienced during Mrs. Mix's prayer in my behalf; all pain left me, and I arose praising God.

I have been tried during the past two years, but the Great Physician, in whom I trust, has been near at hand, removing pain and renewing strength in answer to the prayer of faith immediately.

Once during the past two years my faith has been somewhat severely tested. I was thrown from a sleigh, and my arm was *severely bruised.* In the name of the Lord I anointed the same, leaving myself in the care of the Great Physician who had done so much for me. In a few weeks the arm was healed.

I have not taken a drop of medicine since I was healed nor have I needed any. I take long walks, work from early morning till late at night, and can endure more than at any time before in my life.

I am continually praising the Lord for these blessings, both spiritual and physical, that are daily received. M. E. MERRILL.

———

In the year 1880 I was taken very sick with what some physician called prostrated nerves; the sensation was like worms creeping and stringing all through and in my body and limbs. I employed four different physicians, Dr. Laurence, Mrs. Dr. Sprague, Dr. Vaille and Dr. Foster, but all to no purpose; for nearly six months I suffered in this way; the physicians did not exactly agree as to what was the trouble; some said it was worms, and treated me for that, until, like the woman in the gospel, I had spent all my living on physicians, and made nothing better, but grew worse; the creeping sensation had become so bad, as if every nerve had left their proper places if it were possible, and had gathered in my stomach and bowels, until it seemed as if I should go wild. I could not sleep day nor night, but would scream and screech like one deranged, and could not possibly help it; and then the feeling would be as if they were all let loose and running all through my back and

limbs. I could not stay alone, and as I was growing worse, my husband thought if I could go to
New Haven that the salt water might do me good;
so the arrangements were made for me to go, and
a lady to go with me to take care of me. I went,
and for a few days I think there was a little
change for the better, but I soon became worse
again. I then left there, and came to Meriden to
a friend of mine, and she soon began to tell me
about Mrs. Mix coming to Meriden every few
weeks, and how many people were healed in answer to her prayers. I had considerable faith in
being cured in that way, for I knew no medicine
could ever cure me; so a letter was sent immediately to Wolcottville for Mrs. Mix to come to see
me, but Mr. Mix replied she was not at home, but
would be in Meriden in a few days. I then was
bloated terribly; in a few days I heard she was in
Meriden, and sent for her to come and see me;
she came, and after talking awhile and showing
me the simplicity of faith, she then requested me
to pray, which I did with all the earnestness possible; then she offered the prayer of faith, and,
anointing me with oil, laid her hand upon me in
the name of the Lord, and I felt the power of

God passing all through my body, and through faith in the name of Jesus, the nerves quieted down, and I arose from my bed as if filled with new life, spiritually as well as physically, and walked into another room, and that afternoon dressed myself and went out on the street; slept well that night, and the next day walked on the street quite a distance, and sent word to my husband that I was healed, and in a few days went home to Springfield, and have been able since to do any amount of work; sometimes when I have worked beyond my strength I have felt a little of the old sensation, and I would ask the Lord to remove it, and he heard and answered, and I do feel to praise God with my whole heart, for he has done for me what no physician could do.

> Soul and body both united,
> Thou hast healed the self-same hour;
> Now can I exclaim delighted,
> Thou hast wrought a perfect cure.

MRS. ELIZABETH BAPTIST,
Springfield, Mass.

FAITH IN PRAYER.

DEAR EDITOR:—Please permit me to speak a few words to "A Great Sufferer." From my present condition of gradual but sure restoration to health, I look back on years of pain and weakness, and my heart is drawn out in sympathy for you, dear suffering one. But while you say "prayer, joined with skill and experience will accomplish much," God, in His Word, declares, "The prayer of faith shall save the sick, and the Lord shall raise him up." (James v. 15.)

Now I pray that you may be led to cast aside all reliance on human skill, all unbelieving scruples, and cast yourself with entire confidence on God's precious promises. By faith we may ask God for healing—not if it is His will—but because it is His will as clearly expressed in His promises; and when He speaks it is not for us to question. Several leading papers, among them, I believe, the *Witness*, have published an account of the marvelous cure of Miss Carrie F. Judd of Buffalo, N. Y., who, it is confidently asserted, was healed in answer to the prayers of a colored woman, Mrs. Mix. I date my own restoration from the hour when I providentially met this same Mrs. Mix.

Could I write you a private letter I might refer you to many others who have received a like blessing. If you will write to Mrs. Edward Mix, Wolcottville, Conn., you may learn far more than I can tell you. I trust you may yet be blessed with health, and, what is far better, a new experience of God's love and faithfulness. You will need to remember this is not at all a matter of feeling. We are to rely wholly on the promise, even though we feel worse and everything else seems against us. "According to your faith be it unto you."

ONE WHO FINDS THE PROMISE SURE.

STEWARTSTOWN, N. H., September 4, 1881.

Having seen a piece in the weekly *Sun* of August 3rd, entitled, the sick raised by faith, and as I believed in God's promises in answering prayer, and as I had suffered very much in the past year with kidney trouble,—the physician had tried in vain to cure me, but had failed,—I made up my mind to send to Mrs. Mix and have her pray for me, and write to me and give me whatever advice she thought necessary, and set an especial day and hour that I might unite with her in prayer, addressing a throne of mercy; she replied to my letter; she set the day and hour, and our united prayer went up to God, united as the prayer of one man; and the answer came with the blessing, and I was healed, made every whit whole to the glory of God; and from that day have been able to work hard all day long, and feel as well as ever I felt in all my life.

MR. RANDALL HARRIMAN.

DEAR AFFLICTED FRIENDS IN JESUS:—I have a strong desire to testify what the dear Lord has done for me, in hopes that it may strengthen some who are held by bonds of infirmity as I have been, and while they are walking by faith, spiritually, they are unable to take one step by faith, physically, even with all the precious promises before them. Knowing by sad experience the darkness into which Satan is ever ready to lead the children of God, having groped in darkness for several years, often striving in agony to lay hold on the promise by faith for my healing.

From childhood my body was never very strong, and about fifteen years ago, by over fatigue and deep affliction, resulting in brain fever, I became a nervous wreck; I was unable to see friends, read or write for over two years, then, by accident, I strained the broad ligaments on the right side, causing ovarian hemorrhage, and many times I was very near death. During four or five years I was frequently confined to the bed for months at a time, yet the presence of the spirit gave me such an abounding cheerfulness that I was often a wonder to myself and all around me, that in the midst of severest suffering I could rejoice. I had the counsel of the best physicians; they gave (Mark v. 26;) no hope of recovery, I was frequently entirely helpless; I was carried about in my husband's arms like a child, from bed to bed, and from room to room; thus many years of the best of my life passed away; I often prayed to die or recover. Gradually the matter of being healed by God's power dawned upon my mind.

An account of a wonderful cure by faith came to notice in a paper. I laid it before the Lord in prayer, read and re-read the promises with great interest; and during a spell of much suffering, while asking to be relieved through faith, it occurred to me the Lord needed no help in medicine; He was able to heal without it, and I asked Him to give me an answer, and soon felt a strange sensation passing from my head over my whole body; all distress was gone. I thanked Him and went to sleep like a tired child; in the morning awoke, feeling well, and with little aid arose and walked out to breakfast; felt a strange, calm rest in mind, and gladly put away my medicine; five happy days passed, gaining strength and hope, but just as sudden as a shock another attack of hemorrhage came. I fought it in prayer two days, but did not understand the Lord's dealing, and unable to free myself from Satan's grasp, death seemed to stare me in the face. At the earnest request of my friends I again took medicine; after many weeks of suffering was able to get up, but the *calm* rest of faith forsook me, yet when looking in God's word I was assured that, concerning healing of soul and body, it meant just what it said.

They were parallel facts. I groped in darkness, sighing to grasp the promises in faith for the healing of my body, having lost confidence in earthly skill, which only gave temporary relief. I was able to superintend my house part of the time, with the greatest care. After nearly eleven years spent thus, a testimony of Miss Carrie F.

Judd's wonderful faith cure fell into my hands. Being unable to sit up, at my request, my husband gladly wrote to Mrs. Mix, who had prayed for her, requesting prayer for me; we received an immediate reply, that she would pray for me at a set time, also requesting to have all medicine put away, which I did, and before the hour of prayer I had faith to rise (although I had not been off the bed for five days, nor even raised up), and by urging, prevailed on friends to bring my clothes, and with assistance put them on, that I might sit up during prayer, which the dear Lord answered, and gave unusual strength rapidly. But, alas! I had not taken my other complaints to the Lord in the same faith; they clung still closer than before, till, worn out with struggling often in prayer for grace, patience, and faith, thus losing much sleep, I felt that something else must be done instead of leaving it with the Lord as I had my soul. I took medicine, and, like the children of Israel, wandered long because of unbelief.

A book of faith cures by Dr. Charles Cullis was given me, which inspired new hope, inducing me to ask an interest in his prayer for my healing, left medicine, resolved to trust again in God for recovery; he kindly replied, setting a time which I observed, and was strengthened in faith, able to be round the house most of the time. Still feeling doubts of full restoration, I wrote Mrs. Mix to ask full health for me, and at her appointed time spent the afternoon in prayer. All at once *every* bad feeling left, body and soul felt well. I rejoiced and thanked God. That night, the first in months, I slept soundly, feeling a hundred times refreshed on waking; after three happy days the tempter (who well knew my past skepticism) beset me that it was my own will power in which I trusted, and after listening to his suggestions instead of fleeing to Jesus, trusting in Him *alone*, *I* fought the enemy, and he gained a partial victory; bless the Lord, who did not leave me to myself.

A death in our family changed our plans, giving me an opportunity to visit the East, where I had another short sickness, and resolved to visit Mrs. Mix as soon as able to travel, hoping through her prayer of faith to be delivered from the power of the evil one, who had held me bound by infirmity so many years, not only with the diseases mentioned, but hemorrhoidal difficulty, causing paralysis of the lower bowel, obliging me to use an enema for every movement with few exceptions for fifteen years.

I stayed several days at her place, holding sweet communion, with precious seasons of prayer, feeling refreshed and instructed in the company of one whom God has so richly blest to the recovery of so many suffering ones by her prayer of faith.

She anointed me according to James v. 14, 15; though *feeling* no change, I was impressed to exclaim, it is done; the night following I was awakened with a strange sensation, entirely relieving my body of all weary aches, leaving me with a feeling of health and strength.

I soon left her place, rejoicing that God had blessed me so greatly, and for some days was permitted to testify to my friends of God's healing power, when an unexpected trial suddenly overtook and nearly prostrated me. It shook my faith because I could not at once lay hold of the promises and be free from the result, though never desiring to use medicine or any other means. Though sometimes cast down with fear and pain, I with God's help wait with full confidence in His word, enjoying constantly the influence of His spirit, and have no disposition to return to medicine.

Oh, that I could speak loud enough for all weary, sick, struggling ones to hear, and take warning from my sad experience, and never let go the precious promises which were given for our help and shield in temptations as well as in victory.

About two years ago, during the time I was asking the Lord to heal me, a marvelous healing recorded in faith cures, impressed me that my husband's eye, with which he never saw light, could receive sight; he was incredulous, but I was led to pray for an evidence to be given him that God was able and willing to answer the prayer of faith. I requested the believing friends and Mrs. Mix to join me, feeling thus directed by the spirit. And to our joy the dear Lord answered us with an evidence of His willingness, by giving him partial sight, unexpectedly and to his great joy, and it remains to him very useful. To God be all the glory.

Mrs. Geo. P. Guild,
Portage, Wis.

4404 BUTLER STREET, PITTSBURGH, PA.,
MRS. EDWARD MIX.   March 31, 1882.

My Dear Sister in Christ:—It certainly affords me great pleasure to comply with the request in your letter of the 13th inst., to write in detail my experience in faith healing as relates to myself, and also to members of my own family, to be incorporated in the book you purpose publishing. Trusting that the same may be to the honor and glory of God, and that others who are afflicted, and who may read what I may write, may by my experience take courage, and likewise resort to the same unfailing source for relief from physical ailments.

My letter to you of last December was written under great physical suffering, at which time I requested your prayers, and consequently my experience was not nearly so full, nor written in a style suitable for the public eye. While I again go over the whole ground, may the Holy Spirit direct, is my prayer.

For 13 years (October 15, 1881) I have been a sufferer from that distressing disease, the asthma. A physician myself, in active practice for twenty-five years, you may rest assured that I have tried about every known remedy to effect a cure, but without success. All have proved to be only palliatives. Treatment, it is true, would give great relief, but the symptoms would again and again recur with increased intensity, until exhausted nature would be ready to sink. It is not my intention, nor is it the object of this paper, tó write an essay on the subject of asthma; but how intensely I suffered will be sufficiently elucidated during the course of my narrative.

About a year and a half ago (keep in mind the date from which I write, October, 1881,) my mind was exercised in regard to faith-healing, and at that time I committed my case to the Lord's hands. But, alas ! and alas ! I fell at the first onset with the enemy of souls, and *when the trial of faith began*, and my old distressing symptoms returned with increased severity, I virtually dismissed the Lord, my physician, from the case by resorting again to the use of medicines for relief. I immediately fell into condemnation and darkness. My readers can readily sympathize with me in my downfall, when they for a moment reflect how strong the temptation to an experienced physician would be to resort to those means which his knowledge in the use of remedies would lead him to adopt for speedy relief.

On the 15th day of October, 1881, I reviewed the battle-ground, and the scene of my disgraceful defeat, and being weaker and worse physically than ever before, I concluded to again ask the Lord to undertake my case. My attention had been recalled to the subject by my excellent Christian brother, John A. Best, Esq., of Washington, Pa., who advised me to send for and read Miss Carrie Judd's little book, "The Prayer of Faith." I procured a copy, and had the book several weeks before I found time to read it.

At the above-mentioned time, all my family being away at our summer cottage on the Valley Camp Ground, sixteen miles distant from the city, I availed myself of the opportunity and quietude to talk with God and not be disturbed.

On that day I solemnly resolved to throw all medicines to the bats and owls, and never touch them again so far as myself individually was concerned.

Being in doubt, in view of my former faithlessness, whether God would again undertake my case, I had a preliminary interview with Him that evening, and with tears in my eyes, and a copy of His word in my hands, I asked Him to talk to me through His word, and indicate to me His mind, and so direct me that I could not mistake the language, at the same time promising Him that if He would have mercy upon and heal me, I would trust Him although He should slay me. Immediately upon opening the Book my eyes fell upon this passage in Jer. xxxi. 20, " Is Ephraim my dear son ? is he a pleasant child ? for since I spake against him I do earnestly remember him still : therefore my bowels are troubled for him ; *I will surely have mercy upon him, saith the Lord.*" Could any one possibly misunderstand such language ? Nay, verily. At once it dissipated my fears, filled my heart with hope and gratitude, and gave me courage to come boldly to a throne of grace and ask largely.

Before committing my case fully to the Lord, I desired to have my faith strengthened, and to this end I postponed the matter until I could read Carrie Judd's little book, which was indeed to my soul "as water to the thirsty ground."

The 15th of October, the day I abjured all medicines, was Saturday. That morning the family all departed for Valley Camp to be absent three days. That night I had the preliminary interview with the Lord, and read a portion of Miss Judd's book. On Sunday night I read portions of the Word and the remainder of Miss Judd's book, sitting up as late as 2 o'clock Monday morning. At that hour I solemnly dedicated myself to the Lord, and promised Father, that I would be willing to be anything or nothing, and follow Him wheresoever He might lead, if He would heal my body of all its complicated diseases, and fill me with His Holy Spirit. I asked in the name of the Lord, and with faith, that He would answer my prayer, although I did not feel that the work was an instantaneous one. I was suffering considerably at the time. I rested comparatively well during the remainder of the night, and the struggle and trial of faith did not begin until the morning.

I give these details that the reader may the better comprehend the situation and understand God's dealings with me.

Now observe how soon, and in what manner my trial of faith began. Only six hours after my promise made to the Lord, to wit, at 8 o'clock Monday morning, the postman brought me a letter from one who for years had been fully conversant with my dreadful periodical asthmatic attacks. In that letter was written a recipe reputed to be, "*a radical cure for asthma !*" and which the writer importunately urged me to try. By this time I was suffering greatly; relief was what I wanted. Here then was a first-class temptation, for the remedy was simple, and "sure to give prompt relief and finally effect a radical cure !" See how soon the opposing forces began their work. That letter was written as soon as I had determined to throw away all medicine, and reached me six hours after my consecration. The temptation was of such character that, so soon as I could become disengaged from professional services in the office, I determined to lay the matter before the Lord, and ask for guidance and strength. Retiring to my chamber, I did so, and was immediately directed in His Word to Isa. xii. 2, "Behold GOD *is my salvation* ; I will trust and not be afraid ; for the LORD JEHOVAH *is my strength and my song* ; He also is become my salvation."

Surely the Lord was talking directly to me, for no language could have been more pertinent and pointed. Yes, *God* and not "asthma cures," was to be my salvation; and that "cure for asthma" at once fell so far below *par* as never to be brought to mind again, as far as its *use* was concerned.

In this connection I desire to show how wonderfully God in His merciful kindness has dealt with me and mine.

Ten hours after my own consecration to God and His service wholly, He laid His loving hand upon my beloved wife, in order, no doubt, to bring her also up to the same higher plane of Christian perfection. While at the camp ground our youngest son, in his sixth year, accidentally flirted *concentrated lye* into both her eyes, burning them terribly. She was led that evening (Monday) from the railroad station to our home, only a short distance, with bandaged eyes, and was apparently blind. The lids of both eyes were swollen to their fullest extent, and I could only see the eye-balls by forcibly opening the eyelids. I was alarmed at their condition, for not only were the inside of the lids fearfully burned, but the ball of her left eye was also most dangerously involved. The *prognosis* was unfavorable, for under the best medical treatment the damage to the eyes would require weeks, if not months, for repair, with the chance that the vision of the left eye would be seriously impaired, if not totally destroyed. Comprehending the situation at the time of the accident, my wife immediately gave herself into the Lord's hands, being willing rather to enter the kingdom blind, if it was His will, than not go in at all. Not knowing this (for she did not tell me until the next day nor did I till then tell her what I had done) I felt it my duty to put her under treatment, which I did, but discontinued it entirely when I subsequently learned what she had done.

My own symptoms continuing to grow worse, I thought I would write to Brother Best, at Washington, to come over and anoint us both with oil, in the name of the Lord, and so comply with the requirement in James v. 14.

I was suffering to such extent on that Tuesday afternoon, that the least attempt to move brought on such a paroxysm of asthma as to almost suffocate me. That night I could not get upstairs, but slept, or rather dozed, in a large rocking-chair, for it was impossible to sleep. However, the Lord was going to give me a foretaste of what He intended to do. A free expectoration set in and continued the whole night, so that by breakfast time my lungs were so thoroughly cleared out that I was enabled to run and jump upstairs three steps at a leap, and I felt as well as if I had never had asthma a moment in my life.

Brother Best responded promptly by telegram that he would come, and a few hours later he arrived. But *I* (the supposed sick man whom he expected to see) was leaping as an hart, and praising God for what He had done for me. He anointed us both in the name of the Lord, and we had a glorious season of refreshing from the presence of the Holy Spirit. Wife's eyes healed as if by magic; destroyed tissues were restored and completely healed in a few days' time; and in a week's time she was able to perform her usual household duties.

Nothing but the power of God could have accomplished such a work in so short a time. While her eyes were healing, at one time she feared that *entropium* (a turning inwards of the eyelids, a very usual occurrence after such an injury) would ensue. I told her to dismiss her fears, for when the Lord undertook to cure a person He never made a *botch* of it. It is needless to say that there was no entropium.

As to my own case, I felt so well I began to tell it everywhere what great things the Lord had done for me. But in a little while the struggle again commenced, and was continued with some variableness, now better, then much worse, and suffering as severely as ever. It was impossible to lie in the recumbent position, and night after night I was compelled to sit in a rocking-chair, or else be propped up in bed. I could not understand why my symptoms should recur, for I had trusted the Lord fully, and expected complete immunity from former suffering. I inquired of the Lord what it meant, and was directed to the twenty-fifth verse of the first chapter of Isaiah, " And I will turn my hand upon thee, *and purely purge away thy dross and take away all thy tin.*" I concluded that the Lord intended that the trial of my faith should continue.

On another occasion, my sufferings still being prolonged, I communed with God, and told Him I feared that I would be brought to shame and confusion of face, since I had been telling it to many that God had healed me. Oh, I was terribly afraid and fearfully exercised in mind in regard to this matter. But my fears were soon quieted, for

I was immediately directed to Isaiah liv. 4–11, "*Fear not; for thou shalt not be ashamed:* neither be thou confounded ; *for thou shalt not be put to shame,*" etc. Turn to the chapter and read down to the eleventh verse.

About the middle of November I was so bad I could not get upstairs, and had to again be propped up in a rocking-chair. I was suffering most intensely, and the sense of suffocation was so great, it seemed as if the next succeeding paroxysm would be my last. Oh, what a temptation it was at such times to resort to medicines for relief! Just within reach was a remedy which hundreds of times had given me ready relief in less than five minutes. In my agony, with my Bible on my lap, I cried, " O Lord! hast thou nothing comforting for me in this my hour of distress ? Speak to me out of thy word." The book opened to Psalm xlvi. 1–3; 10–11: " *God is our refuge and strength, a very present help in trouble.* Therefore will not we fear, though the earth be removed, and though the mountains be carried into the midst of the sea; though the waters thereof roar and be troubled, though the mountains shake with the swelling thereof, Selah."

* * * * " Be still, and know that I am God; I will be exalted among the heathen, I will be exalted in the earth. The Lord of hosts is with us, the God of Jacob is our refuge." Handing the Bible to my wife—who had just then come to see whether I needed anything—I told her to read that aloud, for I could not for shortness of breath. As she read, my heart overflowed with gratitude to God as I thought of His great sympathy for me under the chastening rod. Said I to her, " You don't know, my dear, how much good that does me! It is better to me than food to a hungry man! " And the dear, good woman, immediately replied—quoting the same language used by the Saviour in his temptation when He thwarted Satan—" Don't you remember, ' It is written, man shall not live by bread alone, but by every word that proceedeth out of the mouth of God ?' " On that memorable night, whenever a paroxysm of coughing with its attendant suffocation recurred— which it did at short intervals—I just claimed that promise and cried, " A VERY PRESENT *help*, Lord! " and immediately the suffocation would be either greatly mitigated or cease altogether.

And so the trial continued. Remember that

during this time I was so reduced in strength I could scarcely walk. For weeks I at best could obtain daily but two or three hours only of broken sleep on account of my distressing cough, due to chronic bronchitis, on which the asthma depended. The slightest movement, even the motion of my jaws in masticating my food, or the attempt to swallow any liquids, created the greatest distress. In my complaints the pointings from God's words were—"Trust, *trust*, TRUST !" For instance, Psalm xxx. 1, 2: "I will extol thee, O Lord; for thou hast lifted me up, and hast not made my foes to rejoice over me. O Lord, my God, I cried unto thee, and thou hast healed me." Also Psalm xxi. 1: "In thee, O Lord, do I put my trust; let me never be ashamed; deliver me in thy righteousness." Also Psalm xl. 1–5: "I waited patiently for the Lord; and he inclined unto me, and heard my cry. He brought me up also out of an horrible pit, out of the miry clay, and set my feet upon a rock, and established my goings. And He hath put a new song in my mouth, even praise unto our God; many shall see it, and fear, and shall trust in the Lord. Blessed is that man that maketh the Lord his trust, and respecteth not the proud, nor such as turn aside to lies."

It seemed, however, that my sufferings were as great as ever, and I said to my wife, " It is possible that the Lord intends to slay me, sure enough." At my consecration I promised that though He *slay* me, yet would I trust in Him; and so told wife that, " if the worst came to the worst, and the Lord wished me to die, I was willing to die; but I wanted no physicians to be sent for, for medicine I would not take!" About this time, during one of my usual evening interviews with the Lord, after the family had retired to rest, I made my wants known, and requested an answer in the usual way, viz., from His word. Immediately the Book opened at Hosea xi., and my eye rested upon the ninth verse of that chapter: " I will not execute the fierceness of mine anger. I will not return to *destroy* Ephraim;" (the *same Ephraim*, mark, which was mentioned in my preliminary interview at the beginning and to which I was directed in Jer. xxxi. 20, concerning whom it was declared—" Is Ephraim, my dear son ? * * * I will surely have mercy upon him saith the Lord,") " for I am God and not man; the Holy One in the midst of thee." I inferred from this, and rightly too, that henceforth my sufferings would be mitigated. And so it proved. There was an improvement of perhaps fifty per cent. Strength began to slowly increase, but at times I felt badly enough.

But the climax was attained on the night of December 1st. The labor of the day, in my enfeebled condition, told upon me. In the evening, the family having retired for the night, I sat in a rocking-chair being pained from head to foot. As I sat there, I felt for the first time like giving up the struggle. Said I, "Lord, I feel almost discouraged. Here I am racked with pain, and seemingly not a whit better than I was six weeks ago. Hast thou any word of comfort for me to-night? Speak, Lord, for thy servant heareth." The Book opened at Isaiah xli., and my eyes rested upon the tenth verse of that chapter. "*Fear thou not; for I am with thee; be not* DISMAYED; *for I am thy God;* I will *strengthen* thee; yea, I will *help* thee; yea, I will UPHOLD *thee with the right hand of my righteousness.*"

The following three verses, eleventh to thirteenth, inclusive, of same chapter, read as follows:

" Behold, all they that were incensed against thee shall be ashamed and confounded; they shall be as nothing; and they that strive with thee shall perish. Thou shalt seek them, and shalt not find them, even them that contended with thee; they that war against thee shall be as nothing and as a thing of naught. For I the Lord thy God will hold thy right hand, saying unto thee, "Fear not; I will help thee." Surely here was encouragement sufficient for the most disheartened, and it renewed my confidence in God. The night was most distressing, for my sufferings were greatly intensified from what they had been. In the morning, being entirely exhausted and scarcely able to move, I determined to do that which I had often before thought of doing: namely, to write to Mrs. Mix and request her to make me a subject of prayer. The questions which agitated me most were, are my sufferings prolonged, and am I not entirely healed because God wishes to try my faith still more ? Or is the difficulty on account of unbelief on my part ? On the second of December, then, I wrote to Mrs. Mix and requested her prayers, having stated my case as concisely as my feeble physical condition would permit. Her reply did not reach me until December 17th, but it was full of encouragement, and fully appreciated. The evening of the day her letter was received was the time appointed to make me a subject of prayer. In just five days from the time I wrote to her, the Lord in a wonderful manner made good His promise to help and strengthen me. If I had been depending on my own strength in anywise, the last prop was knocked from under me, and, like Jonah, I was cast overboard. If some one had told me on the sixth of December, that I was able to make my professional rounds without the aid of my horse and buggy, I would have deemed him a madman. On the morning of the seventh of December, the day I entered upon the thirty-eighth year of my Christian life, just as we were about to kneel in family worship, my colored man-servant announced that "Kitty" (my horse) "is down and cannot get up. She seems to be paralyzed." I replied that if Kitty is going to die, *the Lord wants me to walk!* After worship, a glance at the faithful old beast assured me that she could not live many hours. She died in great agony the same day.

But mark the result of this chastening. Most

remarkable strength was immediately imparted to me, and I felt like Samson when he had his arms around the pillars of the Philistine temple at Gaza! All symptoms of asthma vanished from that time like mists before the morning sun. I made all my calls on foot, and could walk up any of the hills surrounding us, rapidly and without fatigue. On the twentieth of December I wrote to Mrs. Mix as follows:

" Since the seventh inst., I have had no asthma and am gaining strength every day; and I know that the chronic inflammation of the bronchial tubes, upon which the asthma depends, will also in due time pass away. I can now walk rapidly anywhere without a particle of wheezing. Surely ' God is our refuge and strength,' and I praise His name daily for His wonderful love to me so visibly manifested. Yesterday morning, having forgotten my spectacle-case, which was upstairs, I ran up the stairs so rapidly that our daughter Clara remarked to her ma, ' Here comes Sherman ' (our eldest son whose movements are always rapid), and both were astonished when they discovered their mistake. Wife remarked, ' Why, you are indeed renewing your youth and strength."

Daughter remarked also, 'I guess papa will soon be able to see well enough without glasses.' I seem to be a marvel to my friends who knew my former condition, and I know that I shall not be brought to shame, neither shall I be confounded; for I am regaining my health rapidly, and the work will not cease until it is thoroughly completed. I have taken—indeed, had already taken—the position you suggested, and I am constantly receiving from the hands of the Lord. All glory to His excellent name! "

Nor have myself and wife alone been witnesses of God's power to heal in answer to prayer. We have learned to entrust our children also to His all-powerful hands. We have realized that the prayer of faith will be honored;—has been honored in the recovery of several of our children from serious illness. Our youngest son, five years old, was taken dangerously ill with acute bronchitis in November last, and all his symptoms seemed alarming. Here, then, was a tremendous trial of our faith. Could we, after having entrusted our cases to Father's hands, likewise entrust that of our child? I very quickly determined what I would do, but I wished to ascertain the mind of each

member of the household in regard to the matter.
I assembled the family at the hour of evening
worship. There, said I, on the bed before us, lies
our darling son, your dear little brother, whom
you see, by his flushed face and rapid breathing,
and high fever, has a disease which will soon burn
out his life unless quickly arrested. His tempera-
ture at the time was about 105°, an alarming alti-
tude. Beginning with our eldest son, I asked
him what he thought we ought to do in the case.
There could be no question in regard to its gravity.
Should I put him under treatment, or should we
give him into the hands of the Lord? In other
words, had we better trust to man or to God?
He commenced to argue the case, and thought that
God had given us medicine, and expected us to use
it, and thus make use of the means in our own
hands. He has also declared that if we do not
sow in seed-time neither could we expect to reap
in harvest. But that is not a parallel case, I
replied, for He has a more excellent way for His
believing children. He finally concluded it was
best to entrust him to the Lord. In like manner
each one was interrogated, and all were unanimous
for the Lord. After reading selected portions of

the word pertaining to faith-healing, we knelt in prayer, and anointed him with oil. He was *immediately healed*, for before midnight his skin became cool, his short breathing ceased, and the next morning he was practically well. The same child in the month of the preceding July was brought to the verge of the grave by the same disease, but recovered only by the most energetic treatment. That which before required over two weeks of treatment to be removed, at the fiat of Jehovah was instantly cured. Surely this is a more excellent way.

Looking at these cures with the eye of a physician, the work seems to progress in a natural way as if medicines were successfully used, but it is accomplished much more rapidly. The *Master* mind comprehends the whole cause of the difficulty, faith grasps the promise—" Ask and you shall receive,"—" Believe and it shall be done," and immediately the believer is made whole.

O, most glorious Father, whose mercy endureth forever; who forgiveth all our iniquities, who healeth all our diseases; may all who read these experiences be enabled to trust thee implicitly for full salvation from all their ailments, and by so trusting be brought into that intimate communion with thee, and be so filled with the Holy Spirit, that mortality may be swallowed up in life. Amen.

CHARLES WESLEY BUVINGER, M. D.

SOUTH NORWALK, CONN., February 23, 1880.

MRS. MIX.

My Dear Madame:—I made mention in my last letter that you would hear from me again, after requesting your prayer for me when in great trouble. I am happy to say that our prayers have been answered, so much so, I feel very grateful to my Heavenly Father and you assisting me, although not entirely relieved, but so I can attend to my business, with bright prospects ahead. This day the answer came.

Praise the name of the Lord, a grateful heart.

Yours in Christian love,

C. B. D'ARTOIS.

EAGLE HARBOR, ORLEANS Co., March 1, 1882.

My Dear Sister in Christ: My experience of healing I am very glad to give, and to have it known to all the world for the glory of God. My heart is so full of joy and praise to God, that I hardly know how and where to begin, for the half can never be told what God has done for me. I never had been well since I could remember. I did not know what it was to be without a headache. I had falling of the uterus for years, and my back pained me nearly all the time. I have had the piles for fourteen years, and had employed skillful physicians; some had helped me a little while I was taking the medicine, but as soon as I stopped I was as bad as ever. Last October I went to my friends in Warsaw, visiting, and I caught a very bad cold which caused bronchitis, and was very bad with it until the day I was healed in answer to prayer. There was a colored lady, Mrs. Edward Mix, from Connecticut, who was sent for to come to our place, Eagle Harbor, and I heard that she prayed with the sick, and if they had faith they were healed of their diseases; so I went to see her the 10th of January, 1882. I gave up all medicine and took the Lord for my physician; we had a season of prayer together, following out the directions of James v., by the anointing and laying on of hands, and I can say, to the praise of God, I was healed; my head, praise the Lord, is well. I have no more of those dreadful headaches, the

weakness of the body is made strong; back-aches
and piles and all are well; glory to God I am
every whit whole. At first temptation came in
form of old symptoms, and to appearances there
was need of medicine; the tempter began an argument with me, saying, I would have to go back to
medicine; but I went direct to God for help, for I
knew I was healed, and it was nothing but the
temptation; the Lord heard and answered, and removed the temptation, and I can say, to the praise
of God, I am healed, I am healed, and I have great
faith in fasting and prayer. O, what a glorious
Saviour we have; yes, our God is mighty to save.
When we give up all medicine and trust God
wholly, he never will disappoint us; and I can say,
praise the Lord, O my soul, and forget not all His
benefits who forgiveth all our iniquities and healeth all our diseases. Praise his name.

From your sister in faith,

MRS. ISAAC ALBERTSON.

ARE THEY MIRACLES?

MRS. MIX:—I wish to add my testimony with
others and thank God for what He has done for
me in answer to your prayer of faith. I had been

confined to my bed three months with enlargement of the spleen, inflammation of the bowels
and falling of the uterus. I had been treated by
Drs. Sanford and Shepherd, but after using powerful remedies they gave me up to die. I heard of
Mrs. Mix through the *Sunday Register*, of some
wonderful cures through faith and prayer; my
friends prevailed upon me to send for her. I had
but little faith, but knew that God was able to
do all things; accordingly she was sent for; she
arrived about ten minutes of seven; it was my
poorest day. I was so sick I could not raise my
head from my pillow. I could hardly breathe; my
stomach and bowels were terribly bloated. I could
only lie on my back; my sufferings were great; my
groans annoyed the people in the rooms below,
which was a store; so much so, they would leave
before finishing their trading. The inflammation
was so great I could scarcely bear the slightest
step across the room or a jar against my bed; my
hands were like marble, and as I looked at them
would think they would soon be cold in death, as
this was the day the physician said I would die; at
five minutes before seven o'clock she invited all to
leave the room so there should be no excitement.

She asked me even in that critical hour could I pray and believe God would raise me up from that bed of death. I told her I knew God was able to do all things; my faith was small, but I would do the best I could. I then began to pray with all the faith I could exercise; she then knelt by the bedside and began to pray; it was a very simple prayer; she asked God to remove the pains and all inflammation; her prayer was as a child asking its parent for a piece of bread and butter; she anointed my bowels with oil in the name of the Lord; then placed her hand upon them, and also upon my heart, beseeching Him to make them all right; she directed my mind to the great Physician that could heal both soul and body. I began to have a little more faith, and as she drew her hand over my bloated body I felt the swelling going down. I then laid my hand on my bowels to see if it was really so, and found it to be true; she then bade me in the name of the Lord to rise up and walk; though all pain and disease was gone, yet I was very weak, but I asked God for strength, and I began to walk across the room and back to my bed; she then asked for my clothes, and by faith I was dressed; she then asked me if my faith was sufficient to walk out into the kitchen. I told her yes; she asked God to give me strength; she opened my room door and I started, praising God every step of the way; my two sisters and their husbands were there. One sister was so overcome that she fainted, and they laid her on the lounge; my other sister began to cry for joy; my husband began to shout for joy; my two brothers began to sing "She only touched the hem of His garment," and strength was given to me to join them in singing. O, praise the Lord! what a glorious change; raised from the gates of death to life and health. I am able to do my housework, and I praise God for it. To Him be all the glory.

Mrs. Herbert Hall,
West Haven, Conn.

To the Editor of the *Journal and Courier:*

A communication in your issue of Monday, the 17th inst., entitled "Miracles," and signed "W," in reference to some very remarkable cures lately effected by the agency of Mrs. Mix of Wolcott-ville, calls for a few facts which I would like to furnish. This communication is not written in the interest, nor by the desire of any party or parties, but simply as a matter of pure justice, and the furtherance of the truth. Of the cases alluded to I know the fact of but one.

I became acquainted with Mrs. Herbert Hall of West Haven, as the pastor of her family, in the spring of 1878. Early in the following summer she was prostrated by illness from which she suffered, and continuously, occasionally improving only to relapse into a worse condition; during this time she received proper medical attention from Dr. Sanford and Dr. Shepherd of this place; my pastoral calls brought me into intimate acquaintanceship with her physical condition, of the reality of her sufferings, her debility, and the obstinate nature of the complete disorders under which she was laboring. I had not only the most palpable proof, but from the lips of her physician learned the same; that there was no room for deception nor motive (nor do I believe she is capable of so doing), was to me very clear. Mrs. Mix was to the family an unknown power until two or three weeks before her cure. Dr. Sanford of New Haven took charge of the case in the early part of last winter, and after a critical examination—as Dr. Shepherd informed me, thought relief possible.

A few weeks' experiment proved utterly unavailing, and the case was given into Dr. Shepherd's hands again as hopeless; the only way of relief seemed by death.

In this condition Mrs. Hall continued, gradually growing worse. On the evening when relief came, I made her a pastoral call about six o'clock in the afternoon. The day had been one of intense suffering, her paroxysms frequent, forcing from the patient pitiable expressions of severe pain; these at the time of my visit had given way to a fitful and uneasy slumber; it was evident the angel of relief was not far distant. At about eight o'clock that evening when conducting a religious service in my church, Mr. Hall, her husband, came in and surprised me and all present, by saying that Mrs. Hall was at that moment up, dressed, and sitting by the kitchen fire, a well woman, only weak. The next day I called and found her astonishingly restored, her appearance improved, her pains gone, all the old disease seemingly removed, only weakness, which was aggravated by the calling of numberless people, drawn by the rumor of the event. I have visited her since almost every day; the improvement is marked, and of the most satisfactory character. She is now able to be at her family work all day, and gives no other indication than of a perfect cure.

Mrs. Hall is willing to tell any honest inquirer the story, which she does in the most simple and frank manner. Her physician, who has visited her since, considers her cure remarkable. I have no disposition to philosophize or propose theories; the facts are all I desire now. The illness and sudden recovery of Mrs. Herbert Hall are as well attested by me as any facts of my varied ministerial life of over thirty-five years.

A. H. MEAD,
Pastor Methodist E. Church,
West Haven.

FORDHAM, NEW YORK, September 20.

MRS. MIX:—This is to certify that after a severe illness of seventeen months of complicated diseases, of which time I was confined to my bed. I had employed several physicians. I was told by one that I had enlargement of the liver, and the uterus was down so that it was nearly exposed to view. I had bladder difficulties, spine very weak, spleen more or less affected, bowels in a torpid condition, inward ulcerations from which I suffered greatly. I became discouraged and thought many times it was impossible for me to ever get well. I had heard of Mrs. Mix and I sent for her; my faith was not very strong at first, but still I did believe in answers to the prayer of faith. Mrs. Mix came, and after talking awhile with me, hope was inspired, faith began to take a firmer grasp, I felt that I could say, Lord, I do believe. We then united in prayer, Mrs. Mix anointing me with oil in the name of the Lord, asking Him to give me strength to rise up and walk; strength came in answer to prayer and the laying on of hands, and to-day I praise God for the good degree of health I enjoy.

Yours in the faith,

MRS. J. D. CLUTE.

CAN THE BLIND RECEIVE THEIR SIGHT?

In 1868 I noticed my eye was failing me; it kept growing gradually worse. In 1872 I was advised to use eye-glasses by one of the best physicians of our city. But soon I found I was what was called color blind; printing or pencil marks seemed almost colorless. The second of

June, 1879, I saw Mrs. Mix, and after conversing awhile with her, faith began to be inspired in my heart. I began to see that nothing was impossible with God, and that all things were possible to him that believeth. We then had a season of prayer, and Mrs. Mix anointed my eyes with oil in the name of the Lord; then, laying her hands upon them in the name of the Lord, there was a change in my eyesight immediately, but it was not perfect, but has been gradually improving ever since. I can read two or three chapters in the Bible without stopping to rest my eyes and without the aid of glasses; I do not have to use them at all. I believe my sight will soon be perfect.

Yours, trusting in Jesus,

Mr. B.

Meriden, Conn., October 10, 1880.

Dear Sister Mix:—I am very happy to inform you that your prayers have been answered in my behalf, for which I thank God through our Saviour Jesus Christ; He has made me every whit whole. I have been sick for about one year, under the Doctor's care, still I was getting worse, and I was wasted to skin and bones. I was not expected to live. We heard that you had faith in prayer for the sick, and that many were cured by your prayers. So father wrote to you to pray for me; and at the time you said you would pray for me, we prayed at the same time, and from that hour I got better, and am now entirely whole. Thank God, from the time we received your letter, I stopped taking my medicine, for I had faith that Jesus would make me whole, and he did, and I praise God for it.

From your sister in Christ,
MAMIE RAY.

A neighbor, Mrs. Croft, was taken very ill on Sabbath. I had just returned from holding a meeting at Hall Meadow, and her daughter Alice came rushing in, saying her mother was very sick, and wished me to come right over. Accordingly I went, and found the children crying because mother was so sick; she was suffering terribly from cramp in the stomach and bowels. I asked her if I should pray with her; she said yes; I asked her if she could believe; the reply was, yes. I then knelt by her bedside, asking God to relieve her immediately and give her faith to believe it;

then anointing her with oil and laying hands on her in the name of the Lord Jesus; in a moment the pain was gone and she was perfectly quiet; the next day was about her work as usual. She said, "Let others laugh about this if they please, I know by experience, and I ought to have been satisfied before, for God has healed three of my children in answer to prayer in the same way." Only a few weeks before this, her little boy Hartly was running about barefoot and stuck a nail in his foot; he caught cold in it, and came near having the lock-jaw. He became deranged, and they thought him dying. I was just retiring when they came for me. I was soon dressed and at the bedside of the little boy; he was still delirious; his cheeks were very red, and about the mouth was a clear whiteness and a quiver of the chin; his heart would stop beating, then it would beat vehemently; the leg and foot were very hot and the latter badly swollen. I laid my hand on his head, asking God to let reason take its throne. His countenance began to change; he looked up and smiled. I asked him if he was suffering much, and where; he said my head, my stomach, my leg and foot. I asked him if I should pray with him; he said yes.

Hall of West Haven, and I will now reply to the I said, do you believe God will hear and answer prayer and make you well? The reply was yes. His mother and myself knelt beside his bed, and with sure faith I asked God to heal him now, to heal him for His own glory. Then the mother followed me in prayer, and seemingly she poured out her whole soul to God in prayer; it came from the heart, it reached the heart of the Almighty, and an answer of peace and blessing came. I anointed him, and laying hands on him in the name of the Lord Jesus, the pain left his head and he began to vomit, which gave immediate relief to the stomach; he began to perspire profusely; he rested quietly through the night. The next morning he was up and dressed, and he was all about the house, and the next day was out doors to play. To God be all the glory.

WOLCOTTVILLE, CONN.

---

4 ALBERT PLACE, ST. MARY'S CHURCH, TORQUAY, DEVONSHIRE, ENGLAND, February 9, 1880.

DEAR MRS. MIX:—I drop a few lines according to promise. I received your reply to my letter on twenty-sixth ult. May God bless you and answer your prayers on my behalf. I am thankful to say I can take God's promises to myself and claim them as mine, and I am improving; the sickness is gradually passing off, and I am able with a little help to sit out of bed for an hour, sometimes two, every day, and my legs are getting back their strength. My lungs are very weak and painful at times, but I believe all will soon be well. I can praise the Lord for all His goodness to me, and expect great things from Him, for nothing is impossible with the Lord. He can restore soon. May He soon answer our prayers, and may I rejoice in His words of comfort: "Daughter, be of good comfort, thy faith hath made thee whole." —Matt. ix. 22. Please pray on for me. I will drop a line to you again, when quite restored.

Believe me, yours in the Lord,

JOANNA TROOD CLEAR.

MRS. WINANS'S CASE AGAIN.

To The Editor of the *Journal and Courier:*

I was very glad to read the Rev. Mr. Mead's letter in your issue of Thursday, concerning the cure, through the agency of Mrs. Mix, of Mrs.

article of " W.," on " Miracles," in Monday's number, with reference to my wife's case. In his communication he speaks of one case where he is cognizant of the facts, and says : "The account of the lady's condition was a culpable misrepresentation." Very well; let us assume that he does know the facts in one case. He, in the other cases reported, assumes that there has been the same "misrepresentation" and "liability to error." I would refer " W." (if he believes in the Bible) to James v. 14, 15. Is the simple, earnest prayer, &c., *evidently* from the depths of an honest, upright, Christian heart, an "incantation ? " Again, he asks, " After the laws of nature have been so ruthlessly trampled upon, shall we believe that the Omniscient Hand, which has placed these laws of restriction for the better protection of the *race*, can be so filled with compassion for the misery of *one*, and that misery the direct sequence of a violation of these righteous rules, that the whole order of a nature shall be revoked ? "

As wonderful things have happened, and as well authenticated, I say, if he is an honest seeker after truth, let him come forward and investigate. The truth *will* come to the surface, for it "is mighty and must prevail." He says, "We know how credulous many minds are when wrought up to a sort of high pressure by the assertions of a stronger will." Very well; if a stronger will can cure let it come, say I, and with power, and don't attempt to discourage *any one*.

My wife saw Mrs. Mix Saturday, March 1st, and to-day, March 21st, three weeks later, she continues to improve, every day is gaining in strength both of body and of mind, notwithstanding reports of a relapse, which I am happy to state have no foundation whatever. "W." says, "But, some will say—'Here are the cures, you cannot get away from the facts.' To such statements I would say emphatically that they are not what they seem to be on the surface." How much margin does "W." allow "on the surface." Is not three weeks enough to prove this cure, strength being gained each day?

Now let us see what the doctors have said: Last year, one who was treating her told me he could not offer me any encouragement to hope she would ever leave her bed; that it was a very distressing case, and one which offered very little encouragement to either physicians or patient;

that the complication of diseases was such as to offer no hope of a cure, and added that I must bear my trouble the best I could; he would do all he could for her, and I believe he did, but unsuccessfully. Two others in 1878 told me about the same in substance, and I had fully made up my mind to see my wife continue to suffer, as one doctor said, perhaps one, perhaps twenty-five years, and that there was no likelihood of her being up from her bed in that time but very little.

Since the visit of Mrs. Mix, March 1st, my wife has been up, dressed, and taken breakfast with me at seven o'clock every morning. March 7th she walked three hours in the house without injury. March 16th (Sunday) she dressed for the street, and walked out during church hours. She is constantly up around our rooms, waits upon herself for anything needed, has trimmed and watered her plants, and done some sewing and reading. Her brain is clear, and she remembers what she reads. She lies down three or four hours daily, but is gaining strength and has less pain than at any time in eleven years. She has seen a number of her old friends, and hopes to soon see more and return their calls. Calls at the house have been very numerous (one day, nineteen), and as she is not yet very strong, we have not thought it best she should see so many strangers. Notwithstanding all these *facts*, " W." seems to think himself called upon to caution the public against " paying any attention to the cry of these miracle performers and their votaries which are constantly appearing before us." If what I have heard is true, and all the severely sick ones *should* be cured through Mrs. Mix's agency, I for one am afraid " W.," like Othello, would find his occupation gone, and be obliged to take the late Horace Greeley's advice to young men and " Go West."

D. C. WINANS.

CURE OF MR. PHILLIPS.

NEW HAVEN, July 23.

Liver complaint, dyspepsia, and tape worm; his food distressed him very much every time he ate. He was in continual pain, languid and feeble, and very weak. I asked him if he believed God could heal him. He said he believed God was *able* to do all things, and believed God *would* do it now if he only had faith. I then asked him to pray for himself, which he did most fervently. I then followed.

I felt the power of the spirit of God. I arose and laid my hands on his head in the name of the Lord. He felt the power of God which made him tremble all over; he said, don't you think I am very nervous? I replied no. Soon another thrill went through his entire being. Again he asked the same question; I said no; it is the power of God. He said it was something he never felt before; every ache and pain was gone, and he felt light as a feather. He went to his work like a new man, and has been well ever since.

HOUTZDALE, CLEARFIELD, CO. PA.,
January 24, 1880.

MRS. EDWARD MIX :—Your letter came to hand a week ago, I prayed according to the directions, and glory be to our Heavenly Father, I am better. I can walk at present without pain; I am improving fast, thanks be to God for my recovery. I shall soon be able to go to work for myself. The doctors gave me up the very day that I received your letter. Thank God that all things are possible to him that believeth.

Yours truly in the faith,
JOHN L. JONES.

NORTH GOSHEN, August 23.

Mr. John Baily's daughter had St. Vitus's dance for two years; had been under the care of Dr. Steele of Winsted, but all to no effect. The father, although not a Christian, was willing to pray for the recovery of the child. The mother, daughter, and myself joined with him, and the Lord heard and answered prayer. They came again to see me the next Friday, and the child was well, and enjoying good health. Praise the Lord.

TORRINGTON HOLLOW.

A German woman had been sick five weeks with bilious fever; could n't help herself in the least. I was sent for to come and see her. I asked her if she could pray. She said yes, in her own language. I told her God knew her heart, and what she said, if I did not, she seemed so earnest in her prayer. I then prayed with her, following out the command in James, 5th chapter, 14th and 15th verses. She said, I feel so much stronger, and could be dressed. I called her daughter to get the clothes, and she was dressed, and walked out into the kitchen. She continued to grow stronger every day, and was soon able to be about her household duties.

No. 197 West Main Street,
West Meriden, Conn.

I wish to add my testimony to the many that have been healed through Mrs. Mix.

I had been sick, confined to my bed eleven weeks, with nervous prostration, female weakness, and weak stomach; the latter being too weak to retain but very little food, such as a graham cracker and the like. I was not able to sit up only to have my bed made. I had been treated by several physicians, but without any permanent benefit. My bowels were so constipated they would not move without an enema. There were no signs of regaining my former health, and on hearing of Mrs. Mix I sent for her. She came the evening of the 9th of May.

We had a precious season of prayer; she then anointed me with oil in the name of the Lord, and laid her hands on me, and asked the Lord to baptize me with the Holy Ghost, and it came. I felt it a gentle healing at the crown of my head, and it went through my entire body to the ends of my toes. All soreness was removed and strength was given. I was able to get up and walk with perfect ease, had a good night's rest, and the next morning was up and dressed, ate a good hearty breakfast of ham, eggs, potatoes, and coffee, and to cap the climax, rode about five miles that day, came back feeling some tired, but soon gained strength, and have been able to do any amount of work, and I feel to give God the glory for it all.

Mrs. E. W. Lynde.

North Adams, Mass.

One week and one day after Thanksgiving I was taken with severe pain in the left side of my bowels. I sent for a physician, he called it an abscess, but did not relieve me. I then sent for another; he called it a rupture. I sought four different physicians, Drs. Lawrence, Beard, Mack, and Bushnell. It continued eleven weeks, and I suffered excruciating pain.

On hearing that Mrs. Mix was coming to North Adams, I sent for her to come and see me, which she did. She prayed with me and anointed me with oil in the name of the Lord. I began to improve immediately, the abscess broke, and discharged a perfect stream, and in less than three weeks I was able to be about my work.

I shall ever be thankful that I saw Mrs. Mix,

and, let others think as they may, I shall always believe the Lord healed me, in answer to prayer.

Truly your friend,

MR. BOCOCK.

WEST MERIDEN, CONN., July 6th, 1880.

In accordance with your request to give you an account of the sickness of our adopted daughter Ernestine, familiarly known as Ernie, I send you the following, which I trust will impart faith to the hearts of other sick and suffering ones, and strengthen those who are weak in the faith of that power which God has given you, that of healing the sick.

Ernie had been subject to chills and fever more or less frequent during the two years prior to her long sickness, and had used when necessary the usual prescribed remedies for such a disease, but during the winter and spring had been entirely free from them, and was in excellent health for her, she being naturally of a delicate constitution.

May 9th, 1867, she was attacked with two chills, which threw her into a violent fever, affecting the brain and spine, and for ten days she lay in a very critical condition. Her sufferings were intense, and her screams of "my back, my back, my head, my head," terrible to hear. The physician gave her strict attention, and in a month's time she was able to sit up in a chair, and be drawn about her room. Soon she was attacked with a convulsion, in which she remained four hours, requiring the efforts of four persons to keep her upon her bed. A counsel of physicians was then called, who pronounced it a disease of the spine, but thought her in no immediate danger.

She was very sick for a week or so, then began to gain, and was able the latter part of June to walk a little about her room. July 4th she attempted to walk from the window by which she was sitting, to the table on which her medicine was placed, only a few steps, but her strength suddenly left her, and she would have fallen had I not sprang to her assistance. She immediately took to her bed, and in the evening was attacked with convulsions, in which she remained all night, and from that. time could not bear her weight. The pain in her back had not ceased at all from the day she was taken sick, and when in those terrible spasms, it was seemingly more than one could endure and live. Powerful opiates were administered, but they produced such distress and retching of the stomach that we were obliged to discontinue their use and inject morphine into the arm or spine, which was so terribly sore and sensitive to the touch that it was a most severe trial to endure the applications of ointments, etc., but she exercised great patience and fortitude, feeling that it was God's will that she should suffer.

The evening of August 11th, she was seized with another convulsion, which lasted twenty-four hours, at which time she came out of it very much exhausted, and gradually failed during the remainder of the month.

In September she grew very much worse, and we considered her at death's door ; she was too weak to raise even a finger or make a motion of the head; I could not catch her faint whisperings, except as I placed my ear to her mouth; her mind wandered; she recognized no one, and at three different times we called her dead, for not a pulsation was apparent, and we thought the breath had indeed left the body. She rallied, however, from these sinking spells, and the physician pronounced her through the crisis, and expressed strong encouragement that she would soon recover.

The time passed heavily on, and she was not affected by the medicine as we expected her to be, and it seemed best to us to make a change of physicians, feeling that should she be taken from us by death, we had not done our whole duty till we had used other means for her restoration. Accordingly the change occurred about October 1st. During the night she appeared very differently, and before morning dawned we felt her mind was fast losing itself, and when the other doctor arrived it was only by his strong will and voice that he brought her momentarily to reason. For one week she sung constantly from morning till night, snatches of songs both sacred and sentimental, in a strange commingling, and we could not seem to divert her mind from it at all. The next week she cried most distressingly; afterwards her ravings were very violent, which continued for the space of three months, not exhibiting any reason whatever. Those months of agony and suspense I cannot describe. None but those who have witnessed such conditions can have an adequate idea of her sufferings, or realize into what a terribly nervous state she was brought.

I need not to say that our joy was great upon

the returning rays of reason, and though they
came slowly, yet gradually, we could see that
the change of treatment had indeed been for good.
It was then January, 1868, and as soon as she had
gained strength sufficient, electricity was used with
a very soothing and quieting effect, giving much
relief of pain, and producing easy and natural
sleep, so refreshing to the worn-out body.

During the month of May the gaining of strength
was quite perceptible, and in July she was able to
be bolstered up with pillows for a few moments at a
time, and we could not but feel that she was on
the sure road of recovery. August 10th we experienced a terrible shock in the sudden death of
my husband, and for a time it overcame her completely, but God was present with His sustaining
grace, and blessed the means used, imparting
needed strength, and she continued to gain.

The first week in September I lifted her from
the bed, and placing her in a chair, she sat two
and a half minutes, and every day when able,
she sat up, till the time was increased to a couple
of hours.

Up to this time a little more than a year had
elapsed since she had been from off her bed, even

to have it made. In March, 1879, she commenced to use crutches, with my assistance, and we hoped she would be enabled to lay one aside entirely, and finally the other. But she did not gain any feeling in her feet, through using them, as we expected; the ankle joints were stiff, and the weakness of the whole body was such that even for an instant she could not stand unsupported. After many repeated attempts I felt it not best to hasten the matter, and endeavored to wait with patience for time and exercise to accomplish the desired change. She was only using a small quantity of medicine, yet was obliged to take it daily, and during the summer months had experienced the happiness of intervals of cessation of pain for an hour or more at a time.

The last week in September she was carried to a near neighbor's, which was very fatiguing, and for several days her pains were much increased. While at this friend's, an acquaintance called upon me, expressing a wish that I would call Mrs. Mix to her, but I gave her no encouragement, not even to inquire where she was staying in the city. I had no particular knowledge of *her* cures, but I had never felt faith in any wonderful cures of which

I had read, through whatever agency performed. While busy with my work after the lady left, I was impressed with a sense of wrong-doing in neglecting the opportunity then presented. If others had been restored to health, there was a possible chance for her, and I prayed for faith to be given that she might receive that great boon, health. I sought Mrs. Mix and listened to her wonderful statements, and I was convinced that it was God's power that wrought them, and I earnestly desired her to visit Ernie.

Before reaching my home that evening the faith for which I had asked was granted me, and I retired to my rest joyful in the feeling that on the next afternoon she was to be healed entirely. I sent word to her that I was coming up with Mrs. Mix in the afternoon, and that she must have faith, believing that God would answer the prayers offered in her behalf. We found her upon the lounge where she had lain all day, but Mrs. Mix left her, in half an hour, walking about the rooms and up and down stairs.

This occurred October 7th, 1879, and up to this time she has not seen the crutches, as I had them returned to the owner that evening. Her pains entirely left her, feeling and sense was restored to her limbs, strength granted, which has increased during the nine months, and at this writing she performs most of the ordinary household duties for my family consisting of six, during my daily absence from home, dress-making. Of course the heavier part, such as washing and ironing, she does not do. She is perfectly well, though not as strong as one who is possessed of a different nature. Very truly yours,

MRS. F. G. OTIS.

FAITH MAKING WHOLE.

From New Haven Journal and Courier:

ANOTHER INSTANCE OF MRS. MIX'S WONDERFUL INSTRUMENTALITY.

Another of Mrs. Mix's wonderful cures is that of Mrs. D. C. Winans, living on the corner of Davenport and Howard avenues in this city. Mr. Winans makes the following statement, giving the particulars of the cure : Nine years ago, at confinement, my wife was confined six months to her bed, and most of the time not able to move from one side of the bed to the other; since then has been up most of the time until January, 1878, and during which period she has not been able to sit over three quarters of an hour and seldom over five or ten minutes at a time, and then often at the expense of from one to seven nights' sleep. She was, however, gaining slowly until the fall of '77, when she began growing worse and was taken down to the bed in January, 1878. After that she was confined to the bed, and words utterly fail to express her suffering for the past year. Those who have had friends suffering from " nervous excitement and nervous exhaustion " can form some idea of it. During all the years' suffering the physical pains have been slight, compared with her nervous pains for any one week the past year. Mrs. Leek of 750 State street first called my attention to the published statement of the wonderful cures performed through Mrs. Mix of Wolcottville, and urged me strongly to try her. Others advised me the same, Mr. Bartram's customer included. So I did, and I believe I have reason to thank God to-day that I did so.

Mrs. Mix answered my summons Saturday, March 1, arrived at the house about 11 A. M., corner of Davenport and Howard avenues. When

I arrived home to dinner I found my wife was up and had dressed herself with Mrs. Mix's assistance. She had been sitting up for some time, was not and has not since been laboring under any excitement in consequence of the treatment, on the contrary, feels better than she has in a year and a half, and is getting perceptibly stronger every day, and is better than before in ten years. My wife and I with Mrs. Mix, ate dinner that day together, she sitting up until nearly three o'clock P. M., when she lay down somewhat weak and tired. She has been up and dressed herself every day since then, taking breakfast with me every morning at seven o'clock, and has not missed eating a meal with me for a week. Although getting strength she does not see any friends. The other day when I came home to dinner, I found that she had been walking, and had walked steadily for over three hours, and at ten o'clock when I bade her good night, she said she was doing nicely only a trifle lame from her long walk. But her faith is strong. She says the Lord is the best physician. She prays almost constantly, and it seems to her as if He was right by her, strengthening and comforting her. If this published statement of her case may be the means of relieving and curing one suffering invalid, we shall be well repaid for all of our trouble.

———

NEWPORT, R. I., Aug. 2, 1881.

MRS. MIX.

Dear Sister:—There is a young lady of 15 summers who came to my church, and she felt impressed to come forward and seek a Saviour's dying love. She did, and all at once the use of her tongue and her limbs were gone. She said before she left home she desired to see and feel as others did who came to the light; she was taken home and has never spoken or moved a limb in eighteen or nineteen weeks. The father and mother are members of the church, they have done all they can for the child, and so have the neighbors; a Spiritualist physician from Baltimore has been consulted, medicines were sent, directions were followed, but to no purpose, all have failed in their attempts. She has lain unconscious and with her eyes closed ever since, and I now come to you, in the name of the Father, Son and Holy Ghost, to take her case in hand; will you please set a time, the day and hour when you will pray for her, and let us know, that

we may unite with you; the name of the girl is
Miss Susan Haden.   REV. MR. LAWS.

I replied to the letter and set the time when I
would pray for her, and wished them to unite with
me at the same hour; they received my letter
August 7th, and quickly replied they would meet me
at the throne of grace at that hour, Wednesday the
10th at 2:30; the hour arrived, prayer was offered;
August the 15th I received the following letter:

DEAR SISTER MIX:—God's name is to be praised
for what we have seen; the young lady can open
her eyes and laugh, which is the first sign of in-
telligence she has given, but she is not able to
talk or to use her limbs, but the parents are very
much encouraged at what they have seen; please
set another time when you will pray for her perfect recovery, but we thank God for this; remember she has done more than at any time since her
sickness.   REV. J. LAWS.

United prayer was again offered for her, and the
reply came back:

MRS. MIX:—I am more than glad to inform
you that the young lady has been wonderfully restored, both soul and body. We met ac-

cording to your appointment, we read the Scriptures and sung and prayed, then I left the room, and my wife performed the anointing with oil in the name of the Father, Son and Holy Ghost, amen, commanding her to rise up by faith and walk, and she did, and as she began to walk, the power of God flowed into her soul, and she cried and praised God in the highest. The house has been filled with astonished souls, saying, "We did not know that God did such things, now we do." Praise the Lord for his wonderful works to the children of men.   REV. W. J. LAWS,
New Bedford, Mass.

WOLCOTTVILLE, CONN.

I was sick with inflammatory rheumatism, from the middle of September until about the 10th of October, 1879. I was then a backslider, and cared not for the things of God, but I had tried all kinds of medicine I could get, and employed a good physician, yet all to no effect. Although I believed in faith cures, yet I did not want to send for Mrs. Mix, but I was suffering so intensely, as a last resort, I sent for her; about eleven o'clock at night she came and prayed with me, and I prayed for myself confessing my sins and promising God I would forsake them, and asking him to forgive me and heal me, and, thanks be to God, in less than half an hour I could walk all about the room, and I rested well the rest of the night, and am to-day, March 5, 1881, well and free from rheumatism, and serving the Lord.　　　　CHARLES G. HART.

———

NEW HAVEN, CONN., 405 COLUMBUS AVENUE.

I wish to testify of the goodness of God to me in answer to the prayer of faith offered by Mrs. Mix. I had been troubled with dreadful headaches from childhood, and as I grew older they became more severe and more frequent; they would last me three and four days. I was having a very severe attack previous to the evening that I sent for Mrs. Mix; I had employed a skillful physician, but to no purpose, medicines and remedies failed, and at last, through the advice of my physician and other friends, I sent for Mrs. Mix. She came; my faith was strong in God that I should be delivered; the physician had been to see me that day, but I could not keep one drop of medicine nor a particle of food on my stomach. Mrs. Mix and myself had a blessed season of prayer together, and the spirit of the Lord was present to heal; truly it was in our midst, and as she anointed me with oil and laid her hand on me in the name of the Lord Jesus, all pain left me, and I felt like an entire new body, and in less than five minutes I ate heartily of cracker and milk without the least disturbance, which was a thing impossible for me to do before; and as the neighbors came in next morning to see, for they could not believe the report that I was sitting up, it seemed to them like one raised from the dead. My physician came in next morning. He turned to my daughter and said, " I am sorry I could not have come in sooner, but I have been detained away so long I suppose she has been suffering terribly. I suppose I shall find your mother in here?" pointing to my bed-room. I then said, "No, you will not find me there but here eating my dinner." He turned to me with surprise and asked if my head ached now. I replied no; he asked where I was in pain. I said nowhere; he replied it was a wonder for me. I told him I had sent for Mrs. Mix as he wished me to do. He was very glad, for he said medicine was doing me no good, and such cases he liked to see the Lord take in hand; and, thank God, I have had but two spells since, and it is more than two years, and those two were brought on by overtaxing my body and mind both. Oh what a blessing I received spiritually! my soul has been filled unutterably full of glory and of God, and I still desire to trust Him.   Yours in faith,

MRS. SUSAN B. TALMAGE.

On August the 30th, 1881, I received a letter from Miss C. M. Dean, stating that she had a friend, a young lady, who had not walked for the space of three years, and that she was afflicted with what was pronounced spinal disease by the physician, and assuring me of the fact that the young lady was a Christian, but her faith was not sufficient to believe that by simple faith in the Great Physician, she could be cured without medicine, and that the name of the lady was Miss Mamie Leo, the daughter of Professor Leo of the high school, and that Mamie's sister Jennie, with the Mrs. Rev. J. A. Kummer, and Miss Carrie Judd of Buffalo and herself with other friends, would unite in prayer for Mamie on Saturday, September 10th, from 2 to 3 P. M., and wished me to unite with them at that hour. As soon as I received the letter I began to pray that faith might be given her, and that victory over disease might be hers, and on the 8th I received a card of September 7th, that the Lord had been pleased to answer the desire of their hearts even before they had expected it, and that Miss Leo, on Saturday, the 3rd, at nine and a half A. M., arose from her bed and walked without help from any earthly power, and on the Sabbath walked a square to Sunday-school and church ; and afterwards I saw a scrap from a newspaper, saying that when the lady walked in church alone, there was such an excitement in the church that several ladies fainted; but whether that be correct or not, one thing we know, whereas she was sick now she is healed, and to God be all the glory for His wonderful works to the children of men.

EIRE, PA.

---

112 EAST 126TH ST., N. Y. CITY.

In the month of January my daughter, 15 years of age, was taken sick with chorea,—the doctors said, in its most exaggerated form; it attacked every portion of the body, keeping her in continual motion when awake; some of the time the opening and shutting of her eyes was the only medium in which she could make known her sufferings.

The most powerful opiate known to the faculty would not keep her asleep more than an hour, and then the shutting of a door or a foot-fall would awaken her. The doctor told us we could look for her death at any moment as the disease had attacked her spine and heart.

When first taken sick she asked me to write to Mrs. Mix and others, saying that she should never get well unless God cured her. Mrs. Mix arrived on Thursday at half past eleven; she prayed with her, anointing her in the name of the Lord. Before dinner she was in a moist sweat, sleeping as naturally as ever; in the afternoon she talked quite well; that night she slept soundly, only waking once. On Saturday morning she asked to be dressed. Mrs. Mix told her she must now consider herself healed. Since that time she has not taken any medicine; she is now perfectly well. The doctor said he could not understand it, but looks upon her case as a miracle.

MRS. CARRIE WILSON.

ELIZABETH ST., NORWICH, CONN.,
Oct. 11, 1881.

This is to certify that through the instrumentality of Mrs. Edward Mix and her wonderful faith in God, her prayers, and the laying on of hands and anointing with oil in the name of the Lord, have restored to me my voice, which had left me, and has benefited me in every way. I wish to give the Lord all the glory for His wonderful power, and claim this entirely as a faith cure.

MRS. ROYAL CROSS.

P. S.   When my son came in, he said "Thank God, I hear my mother's voice once more."

COMPOSED BY MRS. EDWARD MIX.

Thank God, I hear my mother's voice once more,
That gentle voice, I heard in days of yore ;
To God be all the glory, to Him the praise,
Through ceaseless ages of eternal days.

Thank God, I hear my mother's voice once more,
Let all the earth praise God, and Him adore ;
Through faith in the dear Saviour's precious name,
The promises of God by faith she claimed.

Thank God, I hear my mother's voice once more,
Let me proclaim this truth from shore to shore,

Let all that is within me bless His holy name,
And spread abroad the risen Saviour's fame.

The promises of God are true and sure,
From everlasting to the end endure;
Ask, and ye shall receive, God's word declares,
Asking is yours, the blessing God prepares.

PITTSFIELD, January 15, 1880.

I had been sick several weeks, attended with nausea and vomiting. For six weeks I could not keep anything on my stomach, not even medicine. I was very weak, I could not move in bed without assistance. My physician used every available means to restore me, but I failed rapidly and felt that my days were few. Hearing of Mrs. Mix's great cure through faith in prayer, my friends sent for her. Mrs. Mix was not with me more than ten minutes when she assisted me in dressing. I walked out into the sitting-room, had food prepared for me; could eat without nausea. I have not been troubled with my stomach since.

Yours respectfully,
MRS. S. A. CARPENTER.

NORRISTOWN, PA., May 31, 1881.

DEAR SISTER:—It gives us great pleasure to say that our dear little Harry seems much better since the days which you appointed to pray for him.

Added strength and vigor seemed given at the very time. This certainly was no case of mental influence over a patient's mind, for he is only a little over four years old. The work is of the Lord. To Him be all the glory! Yours, with faith in the great Physician.

REV. N. B. RANDALL.

———

ELYRIA, August 3, 1880.

MR. MIX, CHRISTIAN FRIEND:—I received your letter more than a week ago, but sickness in my family prevented my answering at an earlier date.

I feel quite willing to add my testimony to hundreds of others who have been benefited by visiting your wife, and laying hold of God's promises through her faith and prayers. In September of 1877 I took a cold which fastened itself so firmly upon my lungs as to render it impossible to throw it off. In October of 1878 I sought another and more friendly clime, and seemed somewhat benefited by the change, but the cause was not removed. I returned in April of 1879, and very soon began to decline rapidly. My cough was terrible, my strength and flesh vanished rapidly; I suffered loss of appetite and was oppressed for breath. I again left home and received temporary relief from some of my troubles, under skillful medical treatment. I remained, however, very feeble, with the prospect of decline with the autumn and winter changes. I was induced by friends to call on Mrs. Mix. I saw her in November, 1879; she prayed with me and for me, and inspired me with faith to lay hold of God's promises, discarding every medicine and any trust in an arm of flesh. I felt a marked improvement from this visit; I could breathe freely; the soreness from my chest and lungs was removed; I could turn over in bed without pain, and all pleuritic symptoms disappeared. My throat, which was ulcerated at the time, did not show as sudden improvement. I called on her again for that, and it healed as soon as in the nature of things it could. During the first month after seeing her, I gained eight pounds of flesh, and in two months returned home, weak of course, but comparatively well. I find just as long as I hold strong in faith, relying on the Great Physician, I get along splendidly. I feel that I have to return many thanks to Mrs. Mix, under God, for my restored health, my increased faith and love to my Heavenly Father. Excuse bad writing for I am quite worn with caring for the sick. With much regard to your wife and yourself, I am most sincerely your friend and well-wisher.

S. S. T. Johnson.

THE POWER OF PRAYER.

The following, regarding the work of Mrs. Mix at Utica, N. Y., is from the Utica Observer:

"Last week it was announced that Mrs. Mix, a colored lady from Wolcottville, Conn., was in Utica. In this connection it was stated that Mrs. Mix came here to treat several invalids, her healing agency being prayer. She came well recommended, and stopped at the residence of Mr. Benjamin Hall, No. 69 Mary street. Some time ago when Mrs. Hall was an invalid, she heard of some remarkable cures wrought through prayer by Mrs. Mix in Connecticut. She wrote, asking Mrs. Mix to come to Utica, but was informed that this for some time would be impossible, owing to the engagements which Mrs. Mix had in the State in which she lives. Mrs. Hall, who was a great sufferer, concluded to make the journey to Connecticut in order to secure treatment from the colored lady of whom she had heard so much. She accordingly journeyed to Connecticut, meeting Mrs. Mix at New Milford, and remaining under her treatment for a short time. She received immediate benefit and is to-day a healthy woman. The lady resides at No. 69 Mary street, and she readily testifies to the efficacy of the cure performed for her by the Connecticut colored lady."

NORTH ADAMS, Mass., July 26, 1880.

I have had a nervous disease for several years, which affected me about swallowing any solid food or taking cold drinks. I have had everything done for me that medicines could do; they all failed. In February, 1879, I was taken worse; my throat seemed nearly closed with a mucus, which caused me to spit all the time while eating, and finally I could not take bread in any form. July 17th I was prostrated; I just lived on liquids until September, when I was under the care of a magnetic doctor; I remained under his treatment for four weeks, and in that time got so I could take thin flour gruel, and tried to take bread, but could not; I could walk a little and ride, but could not wait upon myself. I was thinking I must see the magnetic doctor again, when we heard of a woman living in Wolcottville, Conn., who cured by faith and prayer. I sent for her to come and see me; she came Nov. 27. I had faith she could help me; she prayed with me and anointed me with oil in the name of the Lord; then I drank cold water, and ate bread soaked in water, all in the name of the Lord, and have done so every day since, and I am now able to wait upon myself. She visited me again in May, and I went home with her and stayed two weeks and four days. While there I got so that I wore my teeth, which I had been unable to do for several years, and ceased to spit while eating. I had not been to church in over four years. I now attend every Sabbath when it is pleasant.

MRS. JOHN N. CHASE.

WEST MERIDEN, CONN., September 18, 1880.

DEAR BROTHER MIX:—Your letter came some time ago. I have not answered it because I did not know just what to write. It is well known by all who were acquainted with the exact condition of my wife before sister Mix came and prayed with her, that she could not have lived longer than a few weeks. She could not walk a step, or even get up or down from the bed without assistance. After sister Mix prayed over her, anointing her with oil in the name of the Lord, she arose from the bed, commenced to walk, and has walked more or less every day since. At the time you were here with sister Mix and prayed for her, and laid hands on the large scrofulous swelling, there was not the least indication that it was gathering to break. There was not the slightest token of impending suppuration. The flesh of the tumor looked precisely as it had for six months. It broke the very night following the day you prayed, and discharged copiously. It has discharged freely at three different times, and her system is thereby being cleansed. She is not yet wholly recovered, but is constantly and surely gaining, and we believe that in answer to the prayer of faith she will be raised up, that she will recover her health. She has taken no medicine since sister Mix prayed with her, and is trusting our loving Heavenly Father to bring her back to permanent health.

I have thus made a statement of her case just as it is at the present time.

Very truly yours in Christ,

S. W. Bishop.

I am ready to testify to the goodness of God in restoring me to health after a long and severe illness. My health entirely failed in the winter of 1877-78, and for a number of months was very feeble; at times I was confined to my bed. For eight weeks before Mrs. Mix was called to see me I could not leave my bed, I was unable to sit up and could only be moved in the most careful manner possible. I had been treated by a skillful physician, who had succeeded in alleviating my sufferings, that at times were intense. Both myself and friends had hoped for a cure, but found after any extra exertion a return of those alarming symptoms which were sure to herald such extreme suffering. A friend urged me to see Mrs.

Mix. At first I had no faith; then I began to think of those promises in the word of God, such as "The prayer of faith shall save the sick, and the Lord shall raise him up," and "All things whatsoever ye ask in prayer, believing ye shall receive." These promises with many others, were they not for me if I would but have faith to lay hold of them ? Mrs. Mix came, she talked with me upon faith, repeating the promises of God; then she prayed most fervently, prayed that those promises might be verified to me then; that I might be given health and strength. She then laid her hands upon me in the name of the Lord. I was at the time suffering severe pain; in less than an hour I was free from all pain and given strength to get up alone and get my clothes and dress myself, and walk about the house. It has now been two years, and I am well, and have been all the time able to work and enjoy myself. I have taken no medicine or any remedies of any kind.

With a firm trust in the power and willingness of the Lord to heal all our diseases,

MRS. APPLY.

ANOTHER TESTIMONY FOR MR. AND MRS. MIX.

One year ago, on the 9th of June, 1879, I was prostrated upon a bed of sickness. I was at that time under the treatment of a doctor who had been recommended to me by some friends; after taking some of his medicine I grew worse, and I rapidly grew worse the more he tried to relieve me; my mother being satisfied that such was the case, called our family doctor, one of the leading doctors of the city, who after a very careful examination pronounced me in a very critical condition, owing to the nature of the medicine I had taken, it being too strong for me; he then took my case in hand, but I became so weak and helpless I could not raise my hand to my head; I could not partake of one particle of the lightest food; all that I subsisted upon was a teaspoonful of French brandy every half hour with ice, but as I continued to grow weak, the brandy was reduced to three drops at a time, and that was too much for me. The doctor came twice a day and said I must continue the brandy, as that was all he could do for me, but my attendant feared to give it to me, fearing I would die immediately, as it made me deathly sick every drop I took. On Sunday, the 22d, the doctor came and felt my pulse; he called my mother out of the room and said to her: " Mrs. Cornell, your daughter was very low yesterday, and is but very little better now, but you must continue to give her the medicine; if she cannot take six drops then give her three." He said he would call early in the morning, or if I got worse to send for him. I was unconscious the most of the time. I felt I was past all earthly help; during the night my mother and a friend watched by my bedside, watching every pulsation as I sank away; several times they thought I would never breathe again; then after a while they could perceive that life was not extinct. On Saturday, the 21st, by the advice of a neighbor and my sister, my mother dispatched for Mr. Mix, of Wolcottville, asking him to come immediately and see me, and offer the prayer of faith in my behalf, as it was clearly to be seen that I had but a short time to live, unless God's miraculous power was made manifest in my behalf. On Monday morning the doctor came about 10 o'clock; he said I was no better, and shook his head despairingly, still ordered the medicine to be continued, although he was told the bad effect it had on me, he said it was the best prescription he could give me at that time. I laid as one dead, my limbs were cold, and my breathing rendered difficult, my countenance was changed, and a death-like pallor had settled o'er my features. My mother was afraid to leave me even to partake of any food herself, fearing I should pass away, and she not see me. At noon she went into the kitchen to get some dinner, but before she could eat any she was called to come to me again, and what a change she saw in me; death was depicted in every line of my countenance; she said to herself, my child is dying, but she would not allow herself to be excited, as she wished to be with me at the very last moment. At that moment the door-bell rang, and my sister, on going to the door, announced Mr. Mix had come. After resting a few moments he asked mother if she were a Christian. She replied in the affirmative; he asked her if she believed in the promises that Jesus made to His disciples when He was on the earth, and he repeated a number of the promises, and she replied she did believe; he then asked if I were a Christian, and the answer was yes. He told mother it was nothing he could do to restore her daughter, but what good was done must be accomplished through Jesus, and according to her faith so would her daughter be blessed. Mother came into the room with him, and as he entered what a sight met his gaze. There I lay with my eyes set in their sockets, the death film almost covering the sight. He laid his left hand on my heart and his right hand on my eyes, and told my mother to pray. She fell upon her knees and poured out her soul in prayer to God for the preservation of her child, and a speedy restoration of my health and strength again, with all the faith she could command, and she says she never knew what faith in God was until that day; and when mother had ceased praying I remained motionless as ever. Mr. Mix talked to God the same as a child would to a tender parent. He told God of the promises He had made to His children, and quoted many passages of scripture, and such an appeal to the throne of grace is seldom heard. Oh, the simplicity of the prayer, so humble, so sincere! The very place seemed holy. And when they had finished prayer they arose from their knees, and mother, wiping the tears from her eyes, looked at me, and my face was natural as ever, my eyes were bright, and I looked at mother and smiled. Mother could hardly believe it to be true, although she was trying to have faith. Mother spoke to me and asked me how I felt; I told her a great deal better; this was the first of my knowing that Mr. Mix had come, but mother has since told me about it. I could speak louder and stronger than I had for a long time. We then returned thanks to God for His answering the petitions; I then for the first time since my prostration arose up in bed and asked for a fan to fan myself with. All this was accomplished in less than two hours. Mother said she was not prepared to see such a great change, and was a little fearful that it was too good to last; still she tried hard to have faith and not doubt. She thought when the doctor came if he pronounced me better she would be satisfied. I began to be hungry and asked for food; they were compelled to be very careful what they gave me as I had not eaten in so long a time. So they gave me light food, and I rested well all night and awoke in the morning feeling much refreshed, and was thankful to God that I had so far recovered. Mr. Mix came in in the morning and prayed with me again, and then returned home. Our family doctor soon came, and from the expression of his countenance he expected to see a corpse. He entered the room softly and looked at me, he raised his hands with astonishment, took my hand, felt my pulse. " Why, Miss Cornell," said he, " your pulse is as strong as mine, you are well, you do not need my care any longer. I will give you a prescription for some iron," and left, saying if he was needed to send for him. But the iron was not bought, neither has the doctor been called since, for I have enjoyed better health since my recovery by prayer than ever before. On the fourth day Mrs. Mix came and anointed me, and prayed God to remove every vestige of disease; and from that treatment all the lingering pains were removed, and from that time I have not taken one cent's worth of medicine of any kind. I only pray and trust, and I wish to add a word to the afflicted, that all things are possible to him that believeth. VIDELLA V. CORNELL,

39 Spery Street,

New Haven, Conn.

HINSDALE, MASS., March 25, 1880.

I wish to give testimony to my long illness, and of my wonderful cure. I was taken sick the last of February, 1875, but was able to be around the house until the first week of March. The 6th the doctor was called, I got no better; two days after he came to see me I was unable to sit up any, on account of the pain in my back. After I had been sick three weeks the doctor wanted counsel, one of the best doctors in Pittsfield was sent for; he came, the disease was pronounced inflammation of the kidneys. I had used blisters, which gave me some relief; all kinds of medicine were tried. I soon got so I could keep nothing on my stomach, and would have spells of vomiting every few moments. For days all I could take was ice; my head pained me fearfully, was obliged to keep a bag of ice on it day and night; leeches were tried on my head, and they gave some little relief, but I continued to grow worse until May, when they thought I could live but a few days. Doctors from other towns were called, they all said my physician was doing all that could be done; I was in such pain, and could take no medicine in my stomach, so the doctor began to inject morphine into my limbs. I began to feel a little better, but was unable to sit up any, having constant pain in my back; I had used over fifty blisters, and some of the time would be more comfortable ; I was carried from one bed to another by the doctor, and he thought I would be able soon to sit up a little; I had a seton kept in nine weeks, and I continued to suffer; a reclining chair was bought, the doctor put me in it a few times, but it made me worse. We had heard that Mr. and Mrs. Mix were in Pittsfield, and we sent for them ; they came November 26, 1879. I was then very helpless, and was using morphine all the time. After prayer for my healing I was enabled to rise up in bed, and with a little assistance from Mrs. Mix walked a few feet to a chair, and in about half an hour I walked back to the bed alone; I had been in the habit of having morphine injected five or six times in twenty-four hours, and the doctor said it would kill me to leave it off, but in answer to the prayer of faith I was enabled to leave it off entirely. One week from the day they called to see me, I walked out to the carriage, got in and rode one mile. In less than two weeks, when Mr. and Mrs. Mix went to their home in Connecticut, I was able to go with

them; I staid with them four weeks and then
came home alone. I am now quite well and strong,
and can walk half a mile to church and back; I can
do a good deal of house work, and have taken no
medicine since. When I see what a change the
Lord has wrought in me I feel I cannot thank
Him enough. I can say truly, come all the world
and I will tell you what the Lord has done for me.

Yours, trusting in Jesus,
MARY E. MACK.

———

SOUTHINGTON, CONN., October 13, 1880.

Many instances of healing being recorded in
this book, I, too, would tell of God's boundless love
and mercy to me. For more than twelve years
have been subject to severe neuralgia sick headaches, and as strength gradually failed these attacks were followed by fainting and, at last, spasms.
For the past six years I have been a suffering
invalid, and for two and one half years was almost
constantly prostrated by complicated troubles
and nervous prostration. Sleep for long intervals
was a stranger, and whenever I could sleep would
become so exhausted that on awaking I would
be gasping for breath and fainting instantly, and

the derangement of my bodily powers brought
with it nearly every variety of pain. I became so
reduced in strength, and so sensitive were my
nerves, that the least change or excitement would
produce faint sinking spells, and for weeks little
or no hopes of my recovery. No description of
my weakness and suffering can be given. During my sickness have been attended by seven different physicians, receiving no decided relief. At
last Dr. Alling, a very skillful physician from New
Haven, was called, and I was greatly benefited
while under his care, but at the time of my
seeing Mrs. Mix I was not able to stand upon my
feet or walk without support. I was obliged to
take nervine two and three times a day, and other
medicine, besides using other remedies. She requested me to lay aside all medicine, and support
was removed, and during prayer I immediately
perceived a change in the diseased part of my
system, and could walk about more comfortably
than before in five years. Sleep became more
natural and refreshing. And, as I ventured
forth leaning upon God and his promises, I found
my faith was to be tested, and at almost every
step I met the foe. But to him that o'ercometh

God giveth a crown. My improvement was rather slow, but I could praise and thank God for *my slow improvement.* After several months I met with Mrs. Mix again, and in less than a week I received a still greater blessing, the change in my system became more and more perceptible, but during this physical change I was very weak; yet, notwithstanding, I was able to wait upon myself and do many things I had not been able to do previously. I felt to exclaim, "Oh! for a thousand tongues to sing." And a spiritual blessing followed, of which I would relate, "but the half can never be told." I was surrounded by heavy darkness, there was not a ray of light in my horizon, and I was driven to the very verge of despair. But at last, away, *far, far away,* almost out of sight, there beamed the faintest gleam of hope. Thank God for that faint gleam. It was but a glimmer through the gloom. And then came this promise shining bright and clear, "I will not fail thee nor forsake thee." I clung to this, for my only hope was in Christ. I was then standing at the end of a long and narrow road. Oh! so anxious to press forward in this narrow path, but I was utterly helpless, and while standing there in my weakness, Jesus came to me saying: "Fear not, for I have redeemed thee, I have called thee by name, thou art mine." I placed my hand in His saying, "I will fear no evil, for thou art with me." I walked with Jesus. And most gladly therefore did I glory in my infirmities that the power of Christ could rest upon me. I was then left standing alone and yet I was not alone, and before me was a dark and heavy cloud; I was to pass through this cloud. I was to work out my own salvation with fear and trembling. At this point I remained for several weeks, and at last I passed through. Victory was mine, thanks be to God which giveth us the victory through our Lord Jesus Christ. At the close of two months from this, as I retired for the night, I sank into a quiet sleep, and slept for several hours, and as I awoke I thanked God for that refreshing sleep; never during my sickness had I enjoyed such rest. Just then a feeling passed over me, different from anything I had ever experienced, and just as I seemed to be sinking I heard a voice so tenderly saying, "Jesus is healing thee." I could not move my lips to speak, but from the depths of my inmost soul I cried, thank God! thank God! My feelings were beyond expression. I realized the nearness of my Saviour, and God's power coursing through every vein. And again I was weak and feeble, and for a time there seemed to be no perceptible gain. But in my body I was healed, and as I venture out little by little my strength is gradually returning. I do considerable light work, have walked about a quarter of a mile without resting; and again I thank God that I am still improving and still trusting.

MRS. MARIA BYINGTON.

Mary Perkins had a severe bilious headache, and very sick at the stomach, and was obliged to go to bed. I knelt in earnest prayer to God in her behalf, and she arose and came to the table and ate, and then went around about her duties. Soon the enemy began to tempt her again, and to make her think she was worse again. I laid hands on her and prayed, bidding disease depart in the name of Jesus. And, thank the Lord, it did go, and she was perfectly well.

NEW HAVEN, July 20.

Mrs. Seymour, who was nearly blind, was impressed that if I should see her and lay hands on her, she would be healed. She could not see well enough to tell whether a person across the room was white or black. I prayed with her and laid hands upon her eyes in the name of Jesus, and when I took them off she could see my face, and she felt the power of God. The next time I saw her I laid hands on her eyes again, and told her to put on her glasses and try to read the Bible, and she read it right off. Soon after that she pieced a bed-quilt containing one thousand and four pieces. God can open the eyes of the blind.

WOLCOTTVILLE, CONN.

CASE OF EDDIE HUMPHRY.

He had fever for nearly two weeks, leaving him with his bowels very much constipated. He expressed to his parents a great desire to see me. Accordingly I was sent for. When I arrived I found their family physician present, who had been attending him twice a day for two days; his bowels were bloated badly, and had not moved for several days. I proposed a season of prayer, and Eddie, his mother, and aunt, and myself all united in a prayer of faith for the dear sick boy. I then anointed him with oil in the name of the Lord. All pain soon left his bowels, the bloat went down, his aches and pains were all gone; he sat up in bed feeling quite cheerful; his physician then came into the room and said, " Eddie, this is better than taking medicine." The reply was, " *Yes, sir.*" He then told him he was doing well, and would not need him any more, and told the father of the child the same. I told them when his bowels moved he would have a severe time, but for them not to be frightened, and to rub his bowels but not give any medicine. I left, telling them if they wanted me to come for me. Some time after he was taken with severe pain, and they, being frightened, sent for the physician, but before he arrived the boy was all right; he began to improve and in a very few days was able to be up and out of doors.

Goshen, September 10, 1879.

ANOTHER CURE THROUGH MRS. MIX.

To the Editor of the Journal and Courier :

After suffering for nine years and five months, I feel it my duty to let the public know what has been done for mo by faith and prayer, through

God's instrument, Mrs. Mix of Wolcottville, Conn. I had a complication of diseases which baffled the skill of all the physicians that I employed, and for six weeks had not left my bed only as I was lifted from it to the lounge, as ordered by my attending physician. Mrs. Mix came to see me on the 27th day of June, prayed with me and anointed me with oil in the name of the Lord. I passed through such a change of body that I was able to get up and be dressed, and from that time I have felt well, and all my disease is gone. I am able to walk and ride with perfect ease, which I had not been able to do in nine years and five months, and to God be all the glory.

Mrs. H. W. Lessey,
614 Chapel street, New Haven.

THE GREAT PHYSICIAN.

Dear Mr. Editor :—I am very much interested in the Home Department of your valuable paper. I am a professor of religion, and a firm believer in direct and special answers to earnest, faithful, importunate, specific prayer. For a number of years I was a sufferer, and had spent much money with different physicians, but all in vain, until one day the thought presented itself to me that Jesus could heal me if I had the faith to believe it. I mustered all the faith I had, and asked God for more, and the moment that I fully believed I was healed. Although it is now almost five years since I was healed, I have never at any time felt a return of my former trouble. I write this for the encouragement of my afflicted sisters, and to the glory of Jesus, my Great Physician. And not only has Jesus verified his promises to me in this instance of healing, but also in many others. At different times when in need of temporal things, the Lord has heard and answered specific prayer, and sent the needed things, and supplied all my temporal wants, as well as spiritual.

LIZZIE YETLEY.

THE DOUBLE PRAYER.

A TRUE INCIDENT.

It was past midnight. Tossing in the restlessness of pain and fever, Florence lay on her wakeful couch, burning with thirst, yet unable to swallow a drop of water to assuage it without adding to her pain. "Call my father," she cried in her agony to her mother, her only watcher, who had sought in vain to afford any relief. Softly the mother went to an adjoining room where Florence's father, exhausted by previous watching, lay in a deep sleep. Hesitating, she went back without disturbing him, to hear again the beseeching request, "Call my father. I am *so* thirsty, and I cannot drink."

This was something beyond the mother's experience, that water, taken when craved so earnestly, should distress, instead of afford relief. She felt that some power beyond her own must bring help, if it came. For twenty-four hours Florence had neither slept nor drank. Once, when she had tried holding water in her mouth to assuage the thirst, she had swallowed a little, which caused intense distress, and she turned from it as from an enemy. Again the mother went to the next room, and again returned without disturbing the sleeper. She lay down softly by the restless child, and earnestly, yet silently, prayed that if possible God would relieve her. In a moment came the words,

"Mother, I feel better; I would like a drink."

Too much for the mother's faith; she replied,
"A drink ! You know how even a swallow dis-
tresses you."

"Please give me a drink, mother," was the
reply."

The glass of cold water was held to Florence's
lips, and eagerly and without fear she drank freely
of its contents, and lay back on the pillow with a
look of perfect quiet in her face. Hardly daring
to move, her mother repeated in a low voice two
verses she had learned when a child younger than
Florence, and which hundreds of times since she
had repeated to herself when wakeful at night, to
find them bring rest, if not sleep.

> " When courting slumber
> The hours I number,
> And sad cares cumber
> My weary mind,
> This thought shall cheer me,
> That Thou art near me,
> Whose ear to hear me
> Is still inclined.
>
> " My soul Thou keepest
> Who never sleepest;
> Mid gloom the deepest
> There 's light above.

Thine eyes behold me,
Thine arms enfold me,
Thy word has told me
That God is love."

She looked at Florence as she finished the lines,
and the restless eyes were closed. She was asleep.
Not daring to move, she lay perfectly quiet, with
her eyes fixed on a clock which stood on a bracket
near by. Twenty minutes of sweet sleep, and
Florence opened her eyes with a smile, and said,
" I would like something to eat."

No one but a mother who has watched with intense solicitude over a sick child can tell the
music in those words.

Quickly she prepared a delicate morsel, and
was surprised to find it could be eaten with no
more pain following than had been caused by the
draught of water. The crisis was passed, and
Florence was out of danger.

" I was at my wit's end," said her mother to
her the next morning, " while watching with you
last night. And if ever I prayed in my life, I
did when I came in the second time and lay down
beside you."

" I was praying, too, mamma," was the unexpected and most welcome reply.

" And, mother," she added, " why did you never say those sweet verses to me before ? "

" I do not know," was all the reply her mother could give; " but you may take them now, and if they prove of as much comfort to you as they have long been to me, I shall be very glad; and neither you nor I," she added, " must ever forget the night when *we both prayed.*"

Charlotte Murray's lines so fully express our feelings that we quote them here :

" He healed them all—the blind, the lame, the palsied,
  The sick in body and the weak in mind ;
Whoever came, no matter how afflicted,
  Were sure a sovereign remedy to find.
His word gave health, His touch restored the vigor
  To every weary, pain-exhausted frame ;
And all He asked before He gave the blessing,
  Was *simple faith in Him* from those who came.

" And is our Lord the kind, the good, the tender,
  Less loving now than in those days of old ?
Or is it that our faith is growing feeble,
  And Christian energy is waxing cold ?
Why do we not, with equal expectation,
  Now bring our sick ones to the Lord in prayer,
Right through the throng of unbelieving scruples,
  Up to His very side and leave them there ?

"He never health refused in by-gone ages,
  Nor feared to take the 'chastisement' away;
Then why not ask it now, instead of praying
  For patience to endure from day to day?"

CRESTON, ILL., February 10, 1880.

MRS. EDWARD MIX.

Dear Friend:—Our prayers have been answered, and I am getting well, commenced to improve right away. My faith has been greatly strengthened, and my heart is full of praise to God.

I thank you very much for your kindly interest, and shall always remember you and your labors in my prayers.

Yours with deep gratitude,

CARRIE F. COBB.

MRS. NEWEY having neuralgia on the heart was cured immediately by prayer and laying on of hands.

WOLCOTTVILLE, CONN.

Mr. Samuel Brown of New Haven received an injury while in the army, from a shell, and his left limb was affected. He used a crutch; he also had asthma. He had once loved God, but at the time he came to be healed he was as the prodigal son. After talking with him awhile and telling him what God required of him in order to be healed, he knelt down and as he attempted to pray burst into such a flood of tears, confessed his faults and promised to forsake his evil ways. The Lord heard and answered prayer. I anointed with oil in the name of the Lord and laid my hands upon him. He said, "How strangely my limb feels." I told him in the name of the Lord to rise up and walk; he arose from the chair and without his crutch walked off as well as ever, and when he went away carried his crutch over his shoulder.

A young lady named Adele Shattuck, living in Saratoga county, New York, has just been restored from a paralytic condition, by means of her own prayers. Four years ago, at the age of eighteen, from grief at the loss of her brother, she went into nervous convulsions, and became a hopeless paralytic. All the doctors said she would never recover, but she had faith that she should, and she rested in the efficacy of prayer to restore herself. The other day she astonished her family by appearing down-stairs cured, as she said, by prayer. Gradually her strength returned, and the recovery of her voice followed.

———

The Brookfield correspondent of the *Danbury News* writes the following in regard to Mrs. Carpenter of that place:—"There has certainly been a marvelous change in her condition. Before Mrs. Mix went to see her she was in a very weak condition, having become so reduced by severe attacks of hemorrhages of the lungs, that when moved from her bed to the chair, she could only sit up a few moments on account of weak lungs and great palpitation of the heart. The latter trouble was occasioned by the least exertion or excitement. For a long time her limbs had been cold and numb below the knees; it was utterly impossible for her to stand, although she had made many attempts to stand alone, and had exerted herself to the utmost to stand alone only a few hours before Mrs. Mix came. While Mrs. Mix was with her a great change came over her.

"The blood began to circulate, the weakness in her lungs and heart was immediately relieved, and within an hour she was up and dressed and walking about. Since then she has continued to improve, having no returns of hemorrhages. She can walk and ride, and attend to part of her household work. Possibly the many instances of God's power, so plainly evident to all but those who having eyes yet see not, may lead even this faithless generation to acknowledge that 'All things are possible to him that believeth.'"

A LETTER FROM MRS. WILTON.

Mrs. Mix came to see me on Monday, the twenty-eighth of April, 1879. Then I had been sick and lame for one year, one month and four days. In that time I have been a great sufferer, both night and day, suffering from heart affection, which at times was so bad that I had awful spasms and was in constant pain every day, and I have n't been able to walk scarcely any in that time, and not a step for long months; have had to be lifted from my bed to my easy-chair and back all the time, and carried from one room to another; and when I sat up in my chair I had to keep my feet in another chair. I could not let them down on the floor on account of the pain in my body and limbs, nor could I stand alone a moment. I have had several good physicians, but got no help. I was about to give up in despair, when I heard of the wonderful cures performed through Mrs. Mix. I sent for her to come and see me; when she came into the room she asked if I had faith to be healed. I told her I had perfect faith; she then anointed me and laid hands on me, all the while praying God to heal me. I prayed with her, and our prayers were answered, for in less than an hour after she began to labor with me I got up, dressed, and walked out into the other room as well as anybody, perfectly free from pain and all my lameness gone. Although I am very weak from being sick so long, yet I am gaining strength all the time; after she went away I walked about my room, and went out to tea with the rest, and the next morning got up, dressed, combed my hair and went out to breakfast. Something I have n't done before in over a year. I am still gaining strength fast and feel well. I would add that all sufferers who may see this *may* have faith in God. Send for Mrs. Mix and be cured.

Mrs. G. A. Wilton.

Mrs. Lee suffered from great pain and burning in her back, and her side troubled her so she had not laid on that side for three years. She had caused a rupture by lifting; her lungs were weak, causing much distress for breath. She was under a physician's care all the time. She came the twenty-second of June to board with me two weeks. She arose Sabbath morning to dress, and afterwards told me she had to lie down three times while dressing. I called her down to prayers, not knowing then how badly she felt. I prayed for her, and as I prayed, I felt the power of God come upon me.

I arose and laid my hands on her in the name of the Lord. The healing power was so strong upon her that she shook and trembled, and lost her strength. The tears were coursing very fast down her cheeks. I spoke to her, but she could not answer; as soon as strength came to her, she stood upon her feet and raised both arms, exclaiming, " How strong I feel! All pain and bad feeling is gone from my back, and my lungs feel strong." She went to her room and knelt in solemn prayer and praise to God. She said she felt the power go all through her lungs and down her back; she soon got so she could go upstairs without the least exertion, and could lie on that side as well as ever, and without any of the pains returning.

IRISH WOMAN CURED OF DROPSY.

July 23.

We both prayed, and after I had prayed and laid hands on her, she felt the power of God, and exclaimed, "Glory be to God for such relief."

MRS. BROWN'S LAMENESS AND OLD AGE.

October 12.

I labored with her in prayer and laying on of hands, and she went home feeling much better. She had n't been able to dress herself or comb her hair for several years, but the next morning she arose and dressed herself, and the next Lord's day gave in her testimony as being healed fully. God has promised to renew youth and strength if we call upon him for it.

Mrs. Hart, Wolcottville, Conn., had a severe attack of bilious fever and headache, and was confined to her bed. I labored with her by prayer and laying on of hands; she arose from her bed by faith, and walked around the room; soon she threw up a great quantity of bile. I went away and she was able to come to the piazza and was feeling quite bright. She was able to go about her work, and in two days did the washing. There is no God like our God.

WOLCOTTVILLE, CONN.

Frederick Hart, having neuralgia in the head and face, pain in his limbs, and a good deal of fever, was obliged to stay home from the shop all day.

I prayed and laid hands on him, and he felt the power all through him. He began to perspire from the crown of his head to the sole of his foot; he was better right away, and went to meeting that very evening.

WOLCOTTVILLE, CONN.

Mr. Smith's child swallowed a safety pin, and the mother requested me to pray for it; and in answer to prayer the pin remained in the child's stomach eleven days without injuring in the least; it then came up into his throat, unclasped, and a physician came and took it out.

WOLCOTTVILLE, CONN.

CLINTON, November 30, 1879.

DEAR MRS. MIX:—We have been very remiss in writing you as we promised, concerning mother's health since you were here. We were away from home during the summer, and mother had so much writing to do in order to keep us all informed about herself, she did not get time to write you.

Our hearts have been made very glad by your visit, and what God has done for us through you, and this Thanksgiving time has found real thanksgiving in our hearts toward God for His goodness. Mother has continued to gain in health and strength ever since you were here, and has improved in flesh and looks.

She seems better than formerly when she used to call herself well. We do pray that she may continue well and strong. Mother's case is much talked of in Utica, and here many think her cure was from God. All join in kindest remembrances to you. May the Lord bless you abundantly in your work, is the prayer of your friend,

E. M. SOUTHANT.

September 18, 1878.

Mrs. Emily Harmant (liver complaint) had been sick and employed a doctor ten weeks, but with all the medicine she had taken she grew worse; her side and bowels had been blistered with poultices and plasters, but all of no effect. She had heard of the workings of God's power through me, and I was sent for. I found her in bed suffering very much with the pain in her side, and for some reason there was a large lump in it. I conversed with her a little on the subject of faith and prayer. I saw her faith was good and her trust in God.

She believed He would deliver her from all sickness; we joined in prayer and God heard and answered; peace came to her; all pain was removed, and the lump in her side was all gone; her head ceased to ache, and vigor and strength came to her. She said she wanted to get up and be dressed. I called her daughter and we dressed her; she took hold of my hand and went downstairs into the parlor, where there were a half dozen waiting to be labored with, or to see the result of my labors with her. Some exclaimed, I told you she would come down, others said they were perfectly astonished. The next day she was out riding, and was all right. God always delivers those who trust in Him.

"I will manifest myself unto him." John xiv. 21.

For years I have been an invalid, suffering with a very obstinate form of malarial chills, which resulted in great disturbance of the nervous system, involving also the other organs. So great was my proclivity in that direction that the least exposure to damp or evening air, or any little over-exertion would throw me into chills of no ordinary type, subjecting me to intense suffering for days afterwards.

In addition to all this, I was prostrated with pleuro-pneumonia on the 17th day of May, 1880. My physician, visiting me from two to four times a day, watched its progress with much anxiety. As I grew worse, doubts were entertained of my recovery, the acuteness of the disease involving other conditions than those which usually attend it.

On Saturday morning, May 22d, as I lay in great suffering and helplessness, the beautiful text above quoted was given me. While my body was racked with intense pain, my heart breathed its prayer that God would manifest Himself unto me; and all day between my paroxysms of suffering, coughing, etc., my soul-cry was, "O Lord, manifest Thyself unto me." I could scarcely define to my own mind *how* or in *what way* I wanted it, but my soul was on a stretch for a Divine manifestation.

Thus the hours dragged their painful length till the shades of evening settled upon me; still, with bated breath I prayed for a manifestation of the Divine. My friend and companion, Mrs. B., was herself too sick to sit up with me during the night, so at a late hour, fixing my medicines and my drink beside my bed, she left me for a time.

As soon as I was alone I again began my heart-prayer, "O Lord, manifest Thyself unto me." Soon I seemed suspended in mid-air, going through a process of stripping, until I was divested of clogs and weights which had so trammeled me. I then exclaimed: "Saviour mine! make thorough work; strip me completely of everything that may hinder Thy will concerning me." Immediately, as if banished by an unseen hand, my doubts and fears (alas! how many had I struggled with all my life,) like a spectral band departed, and I seemed a clean child before God, with every avenue of my soul open toward Him.

I was then lifted up and placed on an immense rock, grand and beautiful, on which the Saviour stood. He smilingly said, "Now, my child, go to sleep;" whereupon I dropped into a sweet, refreshing slumber. When I awoke I was in His Divine arms. Then I said, "O Jesus! how I have needed thee. I have wanted thee in my business and in my cares, but thou didst seem so far away; and I sometimes thought thou hadst forgotten me." He sweetly replied, "My eye has been upon you; you are mine; you are sealed." I immediately experienced such a sense of purity as I had never known before; and as I felt the sealing power go through me, it seemed as if every fiber of my being was for God.

He then passed His hand over my face, and a thrill like electricity went through me, and I exclaimed:

"*Why, I am healed!*"

I then felt my flesh, and, instead of the parched, fevered skin I had during those days and nights of suffering, it was cool and soft as a healthy child's.

He said, "Yes, you are healed; you are to

obey Me in all things; be careful, eat sparingly, and follow thou Me;" to all of which my grateful heart responded, "Yes, Lord."

What oneness I felt with my Divine Master! My life, my whole being, was swallowed up in Him like a little fish in the mighty ocean. I talked with Him face to face so sweetly; and among other things I said: "Precious Lord, wilt Thou please heal my dear friend, Mrs. B? (for whose healing many prayers had been offered.) He lovingly answered, "I'll see to that." I then asked Him to bless my physician who had been so faithful to me during my sickness. He smiled, reached out His hand to her, and in response thereto she stepped upon the rock, her face all aglow with heavenly light. I was led to pray for different persons, and they appeared one at a time as their names were called, some with pure spotless robes, radiant with Divine glory, while others, among whom were two of my own dear kindred, were struggling hard to climb upon the rock, but were too heavily weighted. Though the Saviour graciously extended His hand toward them they could not reach Him; for they were so far away, looking sorrowful and disappointed.

I then called for another whom I knew to make high professions; she appeared upon the outer edge of the rock, riding upon a little wooden hobby horse. There was much assurance in her face and manner, also much force of motion, but no progress. The Saviour looked benignly at her, but she was too far away.

I then prayed for another whom I had heard profess much, but she was enveloped in a cloud of darkness, remote from the rest. The Lord looked compassionately toward her, and turning to me said, with tenderness: "Thou hast nothing to do with them."

After about a score of persons had been called for and shown me, I asked once more for the healing of Mrs. B. and again He answered me, "I will take care of that." I questioned why she was not grouped with the other dear ones, with white robes and radiant faces. He pointed to a desert place apart from the rest, where she was walking alone, with a heavy cross strapped to her back. As I gazed in wonder, He smiled complacently upon her and said: "A man of sorrows and acquainted with grief." Though unqualified by words, its sweet significance was revealed to me. As I turned toward the little group, my eye rested upon a dear lady of superior ability, and one upon whom the Divine signet had been set within the past year; she stood head and shoulders above the rest, clothed in white robes and with a halo about her; indeed, her whole being seemed a reflex of the Divine. I asked why she stood such a tower of Strength and Beauty; and without a word He pointed to the lonely pilgrim in the solitary place. I understood it, knowing the instrument used for thus advancing this young friend into God.

I then saw the most beautiful groves of which the human mind can conceive. The trees were covered with rich dark foliage; and upon them hung the most luscious fruit. The singing of the birds, with harmony of melody and rhythm, was more heavenly than anything I had ever heard. I gazed in wonder. A breeze swept over me so grateful and live-giving that I exclaimed: "No wonder the inhabitants shall no more say I am sick!" And with the waves of fragrance came new accessions of strength until I was permeated through and through.

Still nearer to us was a spread table; its covering of rare whiteness was a complete fabric of precious stones; and as it hung in ample folds to the rock, the picture was of transcendent beauty. The dishes were regal and rare; and all reflected the most delicate tints, softened by the hues of the rising day; for the whole scene was one of morning twilight.

I looked far in the distance, and saw the world gradually receding, until it became a mere speck, just passing from sight. Then the rock took on extent until it filled all immensity of space, and the glory of the Lord overshadowed the whole.

Then the Saviour said, " Now, my child, go to sleep." Sweetly and quietly as a trusting child in its mother's arms I slept, and awoke in the morning refreshed and well! I arose in the consciousness of physical and spiritual anointing. With perfect ease I raised both arms to my head to comb my hair, whereas previously to move them seemed like a knife piercing me. I dressed and went below stairs to the surprise of the family.

I did not recover my wonted strength and flesh at once; but gradually and steadily I seem to have taken on the vigor of years gone by, and as far as I know I am perfectly well and very strong.

I can go out in the evening, and am subject to various atmospheric changes, but no indications of chills.

What a change! After nearly ten years of deprivation, I can go out day or evening with no more discomfort than in the years before I contracted the malaria. The Divine Presence which entered my soul on that eventful night has become an indwelling Presence. My life seems inseparable from Him. However distracting outside elements, I live, move, and have my being in God in a sense beyond anything I ever conceived before.

Mrs. E. H. Scott,
Ocean Grove, N. J.

MADE WHOLE BY FAITH.

WALLINGFORD, CONN., August 22, 1880.

Mrs. Edward Mix:—I want to glorify God by telling to the world what the Lord has done for my wife in answer to the prayer of faith. My wife was taken sick February 1, 1879, and has been under the doctor's care since, up to May 10, 1880. She was treated for different diseases, but received no benefit, as the difficulty proved to be

an internal one; the hemorrhage was very bad.
At last Dr. Meganhey, who had spent four years
in the Jefferson Medical College of Philadelphia,
made an examination, and found it to be a cancer,
and making rapid progress; that it was malignant,
and could not be cured. Then Dr. Sanford of
New Haven was called, and after a thorough examination, told me the same; that it had taken a
malignant form, but that she might be made
comparatively comfortable, though suffering many
sleepless nights, and the only way of relief would
be to take morphine; sometimes the pains would
last five hours in spite of all the morphine we
could give her, and finally we were obliged to
keep her under the influence of it continually.
She was growing very weak, and to all appearances could live but a short time. Some of the
neighbors thought she could not live more than
three days. May 2d, Mrs. Crumb came in and
prayed with her; she told us of Mrs. Edward Mix
and her great faith in the promises of God to heal
the sick. My wife asked a lady friend to write to
her, for she herself was very weak; could not sit
up more than five minutes at a time, had no
appetite, had lost forty-five pounds of flesh, was

reduced to a mere skeleton. Mrs. Mix came May 10th and prayed with her, anointing her with oil in the name of the Lord. She was able to get up and dress and comb her hair, and assist about getting dinner, sit down and eat dinner with us, sit up all day, and in the evening rode one mile to prayer-meeting and testified for the Lord of what He had done for her, then rode back without any inconvenience except feeling a little tired. The next day came the trial of faith for the morphine; the temptation was terrible; it lasted a number of days, but the Lord gave her overcoming grace; she had laid aside all medicines and remedies, and was trusting fully in God; had taken Him at His word, believing He would do as He had promised, and the Lord gave her the victory over the temptation. The cancer is healed; she feels no pain from it. It is now thirteen weeks since Mrs. Mix first saw her; she sleeps well every night, has a good appetite, and praises God continually for what He has done for her. After the temptation of the morphine had ceased, it came in another form; indigestion. We took it to the Lord in prayer and He removed it. My wife could take long walks about the town, did her housework with a little of my assistance.   She was then taken with fever and ague; we sent for Mrs. Mix; she could not come, but Mr. Mix came and prayed with her.   The Lord heard and answered, rebuking the fever.   Then she had a trial of a severe cough; we asked the Lord to remove that, and it was done.   After a time she was taken with inflammatory rheumatism, which caused her limbs to swell very badly.   She could not bear the least weight upon her feet without causing severe pain. I sent for Mrs. Mix; she came and prayed with her; the swelling of her feet and limbs was so much reduced that she could put on her stockings and shoes and walk about twenty feet to her chair; it was all done through faith and prayer.   She is improving every day; she sleeps well and has a good appetite; praise the Lord for his wonderful works to the children of men.   We read, Matt. xxi. 22, "All things whatsoever ye shall ask in prayer, believing, ye shall receive;" Mark xi. 24, "What things soever ye desire when ye pray, believe that ye receive them and ye shall have them;" John xv. 7, "If ye abide in me and my words abide in you, ye shall ask what ye will and it shall be done unto you;" John xiv. 13, "And whatsoever ye shall ask in my name that will I do that the father may be glorified in the son;" John xvi. 23, James v. 14, 15. Paul exhorts us to contend earnestly for the faith once delivered to the saints. Elijah's faith brought the blessing, although the probabilities were very small. That is the kind of faith we need to prevail with God. Give us a perfect faith; yes, Lord, increase our faith. Abraham believed, and it was imputed to him for righteousness. We are calling upon our souls and all that is within us to praise the Lord, and we would not forget all his benefits.

SAMUEL M. SCRANTON.

Mrs. Scranton has since died, but not with cancer.

APPENDIX

In memory of departed worth.

THE LIFE

OF

Mrs. EDWARD MIX

Written by Herself in 1880

With Appendix.

.

Torrington, Conn.:

Press of Register Printing Co.,

1884

THE LIFE OF Mrs. EDWARD MIX.

THINKING that it might be interesting to some to learn how the Lord has borne with me and led me, I here give a brief sketch of my life.

I was born in Connecticut, in the town of Torrington, Litchfield County, in the year 1832, on the 5th of May. My father and mother, Datus and Lois Freeman, in their early married life were professing Christians. After a few years father began to neglect the family altar, and so went on step by step so that all the praying I heard from his lips in my childhood was, "O God! let me live." He would say that every morning. My mother was a member of the Baptist church in Newfield, Connecticut. She struggled hard against wind and tide for many years, until at last overwhelmed with cares, trials and perplexities gave up to all human appearance. The family was large, numbering thirteen, yet disheartened as she was she taught us to fear to do evil and choose the good. No doubt she has offered up many a silent prayer that I with the rest might become savingly acquainted with God. I remember well when but seven years old, I felt that I was so wicked I would go silently out into the garden and hide myself in the pea vines, and there kneel in my childlike manner and ask God to make me a better child. But as I said nothing to anyone about it, these feelings would wear away. And as I attended Sabbath school and would bring home Sunday school books, and would read of some little boys or girls that had given their young hearts to Jesus, then the feelings would awake in my heart again, and I would wish I was a christian. But as I went to day school my mind was taken from such things.

About this time my younger brother was nearly four years old. He went to school with me. He was a perfect pet, yes an idol to the whole family. He was taken very ill at school one day, and the teacher told me to take him home, which I attempted to do. He was so sick and weak he could not walk, and I was obliged to carry him most of the way. When I arrived with him at home, a physician was sent for. He gave us no encouragement, but said he was poisoned. The thought to me was terrible that he must die, but the next day noon he was cold in death. The thought came to me, "what if it had been you," and again the same old convictions would come up in my mind, "you are so wicked." But after a while these convictions wore away, and when I had completed my schooling, my parents being poor I went out to service to earn my own support. I then tried to find pleasure and comfort in sin and folly, and as the poet has it:

> "I sought around the verdant earth
> For unfaded joys;
> I tried every source of mirth,
> But all; all did cloy."

My father was taken sick with consumption and lingered a few months, but before his death he gave bright evidence of his returning to God and that God had accepted him.

The brave mother had lived here over thirty years. She was obliged to leave after father's death, and after a few weeks mother and myself removed to New Haven. It could well have been said of us, "Strangers in a strange land;" knowing nothing of a city life and no means to aid ourselves with. I succeeded in procuring a boarding place for mother, and I went out to service. Her boarding place was a very unpleasant one, and a kind friend assisted me in procuring a rent for her with three small rooms. A friend paid the first month's rent. She took in plain sewing and a little washing and ironing, and with what I could earn was made very comfortable. But in a few months I was taken sick. I had overworked. Was obliged to leave my service place and come home, but in a few weeks I regained my health and was able to help mother about her work.

During the winter there seemed to be a great outpouring of the spirit of God in the different churches, and again his spirit began to strive with me. So I would go from one church to another. Still I was not willing to yield, and I had kept it quiet from mother. During the month of February there was a protracted meeting held in the African Methodist Episcopal Church, named "Bethel." The minister in charge was Thomas D.M. Ward. Brother Ross of New York was sent for and meetings were carried on for three weeks night after night. I attended those meetings with a heart filled with conviction of sin, and as others went forward to the altar and God for Christ's sake forgave them of their sins, Oh! the agony of heart I suffered none but those who have experienced it know. Still I kept it from mother, as she had never talked with me on the subject since I had grown up to womanhood, and it seemed impossible for me to broach the subject to her. And I would stop here and say to mothers, here is where the stone of the sepulcher needs to be rolled away. Break the subject to your sons and daughters, you will never be sorry. By this time I was so weighed down with sin I could neither eat nor sleep, mother knew there was some trouble but, did not know what. I would go away by myself and pray, but was not willing to yield to God's ways. I wanted to become a christian secretly and have none know it. I saw others go forward to be prayed with, and before the evening meeting would be closed, angels would carry the news from earth to heaven, "the dead are alive the lost are found and sinners have come home to God." Then shouts from the new born would echo and re-echo through the church. But that way did not please me, I had a way marked out for myself. I thought I would go forward to the altar, kneel down and ask God to myself, to remove the heavy burden, and feel that he had done it and go quietly to my seat again. I did not like to hear shouting and praising God, but the burden became so heavy it seemed as if I must die and be lost at last. I finally said any way, "Oh Lord save me from destruction." My brother-in-law, who now lies sleeping in his silent grave in Hayti, made me promise him I would go forward the next evening.

Evening came, the invitation was given, I arose and went forward, kneeling and silently praying for myself, determined I would not make one loud noise or groan. But the more I prayed the darker it seemed, and that God was looking down upon me with anger and revenge, while Jesus stood showing me his hands and side. My agonies were indescribable. I began to beg and cry aloud for mercy. The last I remembered of myself in that condition I was crying at the top of my voice, "Lord, save or I perish!" I was then lost to all around me, and the first recollection of anything was seemingly a white cloud coming from God out of heaven. It came nearer and nearer until I was engulfed in it. Sin was washed away, the burden of guilt was removed and I could say, "Come all the world, and I will tell you what the Lord has done for me." I shouted and praised God until I lost my strength and was obliged to be led home. I shouted "Glory to God" all the way through the streets. Mother heard me before I got to the house, and came to the door to see what was the matter. I said, "glory to God, mother, God for Christ's sake has forgiven me my sins." Mother burst into a flood of tears and all she could say was, "I thank—." That night before entering I searched for the long neglected Bible, and drawing my chair up to the table where mother sat, I read a chapter, and then for the first time in my life poured out my soul to God in prayer in the presence of my mother. When I ceased praying she took up the strain. I had never heard her lisp a word of prayer before, and as she renewed her broken vows and re-consecrated herself anew to God, promised to lead a new life of trust and thanking God for what he had done for her dear child, the Lord heard, the Lord answered and accepted the consecration.

That happy memorial night will never be forgotten by me until memory is hushed in the silence of death, as now my dear mother is. From then the family altar was erected night and morning. We would bring our needs to Him who promised to be a father to the fatherless and the widow's God, and we ever found him to be a present help in every time of need. We were very poor, the people whose washing we had depended upon had left the city, and we being strangers were troubled to get work. Still we trusted God, believing he would deliver us because we trusted in him. About this time our food had become scanty and our means limited, and as we were sitting by the fireside thinking where our way of escape would come, a friend came in, saying she had so much washing to do she could not fill all her engagements and wished me to take one of her places the next morning, and if I liked and the lady liked my work I might keep the place. I thanked her and thanked God. We had a little tea and a little sugar but, no bread nor butter. So I told mother to see if she could not pick up paper rags enough to buy a pound of crackers and that would last her until I could get through my day's work. Then I would have some money to buy something with; so she concluded to do. The next morning I started for my day's work. It seemed as if I never worked so hard and fast before and about two o'clock I was through. The lady called me up into her sitting room, and began to question me about how I was situated. So I told her how mother and I were trying to get along. They kept a grocery store, a meat market and bakery. The lady listened to my story, then asked me my name. She took a market basket and went out to the store and placed within it sausages and steak, a loaf of bread, sugar and tea, brought it in and gave it to me. Then placing fifty cents in my hand she said, "Sarah, I would like to have you come every week," as I had told her this friend said I might keep the place if I liked it. And as I thanked God and thanked her, I could scarcely control my voice for tears of joy. Home I started with a light heart and a quick step; soon I was at the door. I well remember the lit up countenance of mother as she said, "God bless you, dear child."

I worked for that lady over a year, and I never went home empty handed. The Lord does take care of his children. We were tried sometimes, not knowing how the Lord was going to provide, but we believed bread would be given and waters were sure. At another time when we were out of coal. We had put the last on the fire that morning, and no way to get more. I came home from my day's work: I knew of no other way only to take it to the Lord in prayer, that had heard and answered me so many times. I asked him to provide for mother while I was away at work, I said, "well mother I must go, I believe the Lord wilt provide." I began to put on my things to go, when there was a gentle rap at the door and on opening there stood a young lady with a hod of coal, saying "mother thought you might be out of coal, and so she sent you this." With thanks to God and her mother, I felt the words of scripture were fulfilled; "Before thou dost call I will answer and while thou art yet speaking I will hear." Truly the Lord did bring us through dangers seen and unseen.

So we passed life along together nearly three years. My mother had the old fashioned consumption for years, and at last she was taken very suddenly ill from a paralytic shock. She lingered along a few weeks, and, then like a shock of corn ripe and ready for the Master's use, she fell asleep. Words never can express the sorrow and sadness that filled my poor heart, none but those who have laid a dear mother to rest can tell. Left as it were alone in the world, yet God cared for me and after a few weeks I came back to the town of my birth place, and spent the winter among friends and relatives. In the spring I returned to New

Haven, and from there I went to New York with a friend to live out at service. But the work was very hard and in two months my health began to fail. The air was too close for me, being born of consumptive parents, and it began to show itself in me, and my lungs were very much affected. The Doctor said I could live but a few weeks, and that I must leave the city. I did so, and came out to my sister's in Goshen, Conn. The doctor gave me some tincture of barks; and by dieting and getting fresh air, in two months I was able to go out to service again.

The Spring following I was married, and as we had little ones added to our family and as they sickened and died, my sorrows and care and anxiety so wore upon me that my health began to fail me again. During these years since my mother's death I had been indifferent and cold spiritually. Still I dared not retire without praying. As I look back I see how much the Lord has done for me. My husband had once been a professing Christian, and he, too, had wandered from God. So I would pray for him that he might come back to the Father's House, but my example was not sufficient to draw him to Christ, so I could only pray; but the Lord heard and answered; and by searching the word of God we changed our views and became Adventists. We were both baptized by immersion, and so we went heart and hand together, but my children sickened and died one after another, until the last lovely one sleeps until that great gathering morning. It would be my last thought at night and the first thought in the morning, "Oh, children." I had been impressed that God wanted me to do something more for him than I had ever done. Some text of scripture would come to my mind, and I would be led to write on that subject: passage after passage of scripture would come so vivid and plain to me, and I would get the Concordance and Bible, and found I had got the verse almost exact. But as I was very much engaged dress making, I drove the thought from my mind as much as possible.

One morning as I awoke, the loss of my children came into my mind, and the next thought like a voice speaking to me said, "Go work to-day in my vineyard." The voice was unlike anything I had ever heard before. There seemed to be such a compelling power accompanying it that I could not resist it. I tried to cast aside the conviction by saying it was all imagination, but the words followed me day and night, "Go work in my vineyard." Then I began to plead with the Lord that I was unworthy; that I was illiterate; that I had no talent; but the same words followed me. I told Him my health was poor and memory very short, that I was insufficient in every way. Still the same persistent, urgent call. I have walked the floor for hours, begging that the cup might pass until it was shown me plainly that I should be lost unless I took up the cross. I felt like absenting myself from meeting, and like being alone. Bro. Beemein one Sabbath after meeting (I suppose my looks betrayed me, for I had been weeping,) asked me what was the trouble. I told him I did not know, but the Spirit of God rebuked me for saying thus then. I said "I do know; I don't yield." Bro. B. said "Let us have a word of prayer, and whatever is the trouble yield to God." We knelt in prayer. I there promised God I would take up the cross, heavy as it was, if He would only help me. Soon Bro. Beemein and I practiced singing some new pieces we wanted to learn. When he had gone, I thought I would play them over on the piano, so as to get them perfect, and as I took the book the first place that I opened to was headed "Go work to-day in my vineyard." I closed the book, the words were like a nail driven in a sure place. Still I asked for a plainer showing; and as I retired at night I asked God to give me some greater evidence, and I would obey. As I fell asleep—it seemed almost like a vision to me—a cloud in the form of a full moon, very large, and in it three of the most lovely faces I ever beheld. It came to me in a moment, "These are Faith, Hope and

Charity; take them with you." When I awoke I seemed so happy I said, "Lord, I will believe." But after awhile I got into Doubting Castle again, and was so tempted and tried about it, fearing it might not be of the Lord after all. At last I came to God once more, and asked him to give me one more sign and I would ask for no more. In fact I dared not, and after retiring, as my head was resting upon the pillow, I breathed out my whole heart's desire to God, asking him this once, "Lord, give me a bright evidence that thou has called me to work in thy vineyard." Then I felt such an assurance that he would grant this request that during the dark watches of the night it appeared as if I was lifted out of myself as it were, and I could truly say out of self into Christ. In the east there appeared a cloud of fire, its form as a powder horn, but very large. I seemingly was up in mid air, and while gazing with wonder and astonishment at the scene, it burst, and the eastern horizon was filled with stars of fire. Soon they began to change to color of gold, and then to form into crowns; and as crowns were formed they began to come towards me as if carried by a soft, gentle wind. The first, second and third passed slowly by. I did not seem to feel disappointed, for I was sure one was for me, and the fourth came and stopped at my side. It opened, and closed me up in it. Oh, the glory! tongue can never tell it, pen can never express it—I was so filled with the glory of God! I shouted and praised God until I awoke my husband. He shook and awoke me, saying, "Sarah, what is the matter?" All the reply I could give for some time was: "Glory to God! Glory to God!" I said to myself, Lord, it is enough. I felt to say,

> Jesus, I my cross will take,
> All to leave and follow thee;
> All things else I will forsake,
> Thou from hence my all shall be.

The Lord opened the way and I obeyed, and He has blessed the labors. Some of the time my health has been quite poor. I have been to fill an appointment when I would be obliged to lie down before I started, and when I stood up to read the first hymn would have to take hold of a chair or table, for I was so sick and weak I could not stand without some support. But the Lord always kept and strengthened me.

On the 19th December, 1877, I was healed by faith and prayer and the laying on of hands by Bro. Ethan O. Allen, of Springfield, Mass., one who has the gift of healing. The Lord works mightily through him. And God in His goodness and mercy has blessed me with others, with this blessed boon, the gift of faith, and the healing by the laying on of hands and the prayer of faith. How many, God only knows, have been benefited through unworthy me. Eternity itself can only reveal the numbers.

Many are the fiery darts that are continually hurled at me, but with the shield of faith they cannot injure. The tongue of the slanderer has been sharpened against me, but God takes care of His cause, and there is no weapon formed by Satan against God's children that shall prosper. It is not only the world's people that I have to contend with, for I find that many of them believe that if one of God's promises are true they all must be; but I find great opposition among those that call themselves Christians, those that walk to the Church of God with me and say "Sister." Some of them turn a cold shoulder, but the Lord knows the way I take, and when he has tried me, I shall come forth as gold.

By the grace of God I shall stand, and having done all, stand with my loins girt about with truth, my lamp trimmed and burning, that when Christ who is the believers' life shall appear, then, and not until then, I expect to appear with Him in glory, and hear "Well done!" and then enter in. I had rather wear out in the vineyard of my Master than to rust out in idleness.

I do believe there is a crown laid up for me; and there will be some stars to deck my crown with in the day of Christ's coming.

May the blessing of God rest upon all who shall read of my imperfect life, is the prayer of unworthy me. Amen.

MRS. EDWARD M. MIX.

Appendix

Mrs. Edward Mix died on Monday, April 14, 1884. The funeral services were held the next Wednesday, Rev. Mr. Burbank, officiating. A large number of brethren and sisters were present, some coming from other states. I have thought it best to write an account of her closing hours.

For some days previous to my dear wife's decease I stayed with her night and day. She did not like to have me go out of her sight, but said that she felt so much better when I was with her. She did not converse as freely as before, but always joined with me in our family devotions, morning and evening, and always seemed to enjoy the refreshing season that we used to have that came from the presence of the Lord. Her faith seemed strong, and her trust firm unto the end. For a few days before her death she did not like to have anyone to come into her room, except a good sister in the Lord and a kind neighbor. Yet she would converse freely with me on the subject of faith; and when she felt badly she would pray, and ask me to pray for her, and the Lord would always send relief, and she would praise him for his goodness. The Lord would often send his Holy Spirit upon her after she had retired. Sometimes it seemed to exhaust her in getting ready to retire, and to put her out of breath. Then she would begin praying, and the Lord would send his power upon her so as to pervade her entire being, and then she would praise the Lord and be so happy!

Mrs. Mix wrote some up to a few days previous to her death. She had three rocking chairs, and when tired would change from one to the other. Sunday previous to her death she would have spells of filling up. I saw that she was feeling worse, and that there was a rising in the throat. She spoke to me and said, "Edward, I wish that you would sit in another chair so that I can sit in your lap." I did so, and she came, and then said that she was not afraid to die if the Lord had got through with her. But as many suffering ones as there were that needed help, it did not seem to her as though the Lord *had* got through with her. She said, "Can it be possible that God has answered my prayer so many times in behalf of others, and taken them out of the very jaws of death?" "Yes," she added, "even when they have been dying; and now must I fall under the cold and icy hand of death: it don't seem possible." Oh! I never can forget the struggle of those solemn moments! How that dear one called upon Jesus! Her prayer was heard, and such a baptism of power fell upon us both! She shouted and praised God. The death rattle was driven back entirely, so to all human appearance the victory was won. She said everything was different, and was wonderfully happy. The power pervaded her entire being, and it came upon me copiously. I laid my hands on her in the name of the Lord Jesus Christ, and the Holy Spirit flowed so freely with its strengthening and refreshing effects that she got up and walked, and said that she felt so much stronger she claimed healing. She was wonderfully blest. The Lord is witness. It always seemed that if we had held on to that blessing, the work was done. It seems to me that she made a mistake in one particular, and this is the point: Jesus says, "What things soever ye desire when ye pray, believe that ye receive them, and ye shall have them." I believe that she thought she was healed, and that she was if we had held to that point without wavering.

Another Sunday morning Mrs. Mix was feeling quite poorly, and as a brother was coming to our place to preach who prays with the sick—and the Lord has often blessed his labors in that direction—I left word to have him come and pray with my wife after meeting. After afternoon service he came, and with him a sister who also prays with the sick. I told them that the Lord had wonderfully blessed us, and especially my dear wife. Of course my wife was weak, and I suppose that she thought the brother would feel slighted if she did not ask him to pray with her, seeing she had sent to him before. But this is the point I wish to make plain for the benefit of those that look to Jesus for healing. She asked the brother to pray with her, or said we better have a season of prayer. Now, if the Lord had done the work before, it was not necessary to ask the brother to pray for the Lord to do what he had already done. Here is where it looks to me as though a doubt came in: it was an admission that the work was not done. The brother and sister prayed, the Spirit came on them, and they laid hands on her in the name of the Lord Jesus; but instead of giving her strength and power, she told me it seemed to take every bit of strength from her that she had. One might say, how is this? Jesus said, "I perceive that virtue has gone out of me," and the point I wish to make plain is; it seemed instead of their imparting to her virtue, they took the virtue from her that the Lord had previously imparted, or else they imparted so much that it overpowered and made her weaker instead of stronger. Jesus said; "The spirit is willing but the flesh is weak." Mark 11th, 23; And Jesus saith unto them, have faith in God;

"For verily I say unto you, that whosoever shall say unto this mountain, Be thou removed and be thou cast into the sea and shall not doubt in his heart, but shall believe that those things which he saith shall come to pass, he shall have whatsoever he saith."

I wish to say that a few days previous to this time Bro. E. O. Allen of Springfield, Mass., whom the Lord used as an instrument in the healing of Mrs. Mix December 19th, 1877, called and prayed with her and there was a great change in many particulars for the better, but she did not seem to gain her strength as at other times when she had been prayed with. But the secret of the whole was here, her work was done. The Lord showed me, as near as I can remember, about four years previous to my wife's death, that she was not going to live, and it seems to me now that I had ought to have realized it more fully. I did at different times but she had such faith that seemed to know no bounds, that when to all human appearance she could not live but a short time, we would unite in prayer together and the Lord would hear and answer and bless her for the time being. Then she might start and travel off, from three to five hundred miles, preach perhaps night after night, labor with the sick until ten or eleven o'clock at night, then go to her room and raise blood, then the next day go at the same work again. She seemed to be moved by an unseen power. If she could write to some sick one, or pray for them, then she was happy.

Mrs. Mix had a female prayer meeting that she sustained for years when at home. Finally the other sisters appeared to lose their interest; which made her heart sad. But this did not daunt her courage in the least, every Wednesday when at home at half past two she would pray for the sick. Letters would come in from the different states, saying, "I was healed at that hour you prayed for me." Then her cup of joy would be full, and often run over.

The Lord showed me the different changes that my wife would pass through until she fell asleep in Jesus. I think about two years previous to her death, we wrote to Bro. Allen to pray for her. He did so, and the Lord showed him that her work was almost done. He sat down and wrote her a letter, saying: "Sister Mix, you will not be surprised," or words to that effect, "that your work is about done." Yet she would not listen to that, but seemed to take hold of God with such unwavering faith and confidence, and she gained so rapidly that Bro. Allen said himself that he believed the Lord was going to let her live. But God makes no mistakes; He knows best. I laid her away in deep sadness, but not without hope in my breast. I will join her in gladness, and enter the heavenly rest. He gave, he took, he will restore: he doeth all things well.

The night previous to her death, Mrs. Mix did not seem to rest as well as usual. She would sit up in the rocking chair awhile, and then want to lie down. Towards morning she appeared to be easier. We had a season of prayer, and then she wanted to be dressed, but before she could be, she had to give up and lie down exhausted. It was the first time I ever saw her yield since she began the life of faith. At, I should think, about ten o'clock, she asked me to pray for her. I did this, and the Lord blessed her, and she said, "I must get right up." She rose, and with a little assistance walked to the chair, sat a little while, and then said, "I will lie down." This was the last time that my wife ever sat up. She had spells of not breathing easy. A little while before she died, there came a period of distress, and she asked me to pray for her, which I did, and again she began to breathe easier. She asked me to sing something, and then looked up at me and said, "you need not sing any funeral dirge either." So I sang,

> "She only touched the hem of his garment,
> As to his side she stole."

She seemed to enjoy it very much. I saw the lamp of life was about to be extinguished. There was no more distress after I prayed for her, but her breath grew shorter. I lifted up her hand and held it. She spoke to me and said, "I am not dying; the Spirit of the Lord is upon me." And so it was, for I felt its blessed presence also. And so the dear one breathed out her last breath without knowing the enemy of all mankind was there.

> "She sleeps in Jesus, blessed sleep,
> From which none ever wake to weep."

E. M. Mix.